40p

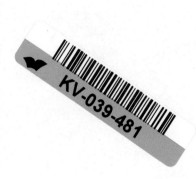

KV-039-481

EXAMINING DOCTORS

Examining Doctors

Medicine in the 1990s

Donald Gould

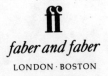

faber and faber

LONDON · BOSTON

First published in 1991
by Faber and Faber Limited
3 Queen Square, London WC1N 3AU

Photoset by Wilmaset, Birkenhead, Wirral
Printed in Great Britain by
Clays Ltd, St Ives plc.

A CIP record for this book is available from the British Library
ISBN 0–571–14360–1

To my wife

Contents

Preface

What are doctors for? What sort of people are they? How do they view their role in society and how do they set about fulfilling that role? How are they trained? How are they controlled? What do their customers think of the profession and what does the profession think of its customers? What is the relationship between medicine and the State? What will the doctors of the twenty-first century be like?

Examining Doctors is intended to provide some of the answers to these questions. It is not an account of modern medical techniques, nor of the National Health Service, although both these topics surface frequently in its pages. It is, instead, an attempt to present a picture of the medical profession and of the men and women who make it up.

To help myself get as near as may be to the truth of the matter I have spent an hour or so with a tape recorder in conversation with each of a number of people who are in some way concerned with the medical scene. What they had to say has informed and shaped my text, and to that extent it is their book.

There is a general impression abroad that doctors (just like the members of other professions) are engaged, as Bernard Shaw put it, in a conspiracy against the laity, and that, in particular, they tend to close ranks and clam up in the face of any criticisms or complaints from patients or anybody else outside the club. Therefore, in thanking those who agreed to speak to me (and only one doctor amongst my targeted respondents turned me down), I am happy to report that I found a remarkable willingness to acknowledge and discuss shortcomings, and an eagerness to examine and, when necessary, modify established attitudes and practices in an effort to make the doctor–patient relationship a more open, fruitful and mutually rewarding partnership.

People Interviewed

The following people kindly agreed to be interviewed by me, and their comments are recorded throughout the book. (Job descriptions are those applying at the time of interview.)

Nick Bosanquet Professor of Health Policy, University of London
Derek Cracknell GP and Chairman, Cambridgeshire Family Practitioner Committee
Joe Collier Clinical pharmacologist, St George's Hospital, London
Ellis Downes Newly qualified Junior Hospital Doctor, Leicester
Sir Terence English Heart surgeon and President, Royal College of Surgeons of England
Raanan Gillon Director, Imperial College of Science and Technology Health Service and Editor, *Journal of Medical Ethics*
Bill Grove Final year student, Royal Free Hospital, London
Sir Robert Kilpatrick President, General Medical Council
James Malone-Lee Consultant geriatrician, University College Hospital, London
John Marks GP and Chairman of Council, British Medical Association
Margaret Martin Secretary, Cambridge Community Health Council
Rabbi Julia Neuberger Chairperson, Patients Association
David Owen Politician and sometime Health Minister
David Ryde GP, Beckenham, Kent
Barry Salter Administrator, Cambridgeshire Family Practitioner Committee
Wendy Savage Consultant obstetrician, London Hospital
George Teeling Smith Director, Office of Health Economics

1 The Problem

In 1977 the World Health Organization adopted a war cry, 'Health for All by the Year 2000', which has become a constantly repeated affirmation of that institution's grand strategy.

WHO's ambitious (many would say fanciful) stated goal is not just the worldwide containment of identifiable, distressing, disabling and possibly mortal disease by the turn of the century, but aims to give people everywhere 'a positive sense of health so that they can make full use of their physical, mental and emotional capacities'.

This ideal is not new. Juvenal wrote of the common need for *mens sana in corpore sano* some 2,000 years ago. But what must be done to achieve such a universal state of well-being?

Given a couple of millennia to act upon the Roman satirist's aphorism, the doctors haven't made much of an impact.

Medical scientists and practitioners have very recently achieved remarkable successes in eliminating or reducing the incidence of *some* diseases, such as smallpox and diphtheria, and in curing or controlling others, like diabetes and many bacterial infections. But millions of people still die before their time, and, despite the 'therapeutic revolution' which began some fifty years ago, the 'sickness rate' in developed nations, whose citizens have access to the best of modern medical care, has hardly altered. Indeed, in Britain the time lost from work due to sickness has actually increased, nationwide, by a prodigious 25 per cent since the NHS was established.

However, while the incidence of ill health has shown small change (an increase in absenteeism does not necessarily mean that more people suffer truly disabling afflictions more often than before), there has been a marked alteration in the pattern of disease. Conditions 'conquered' have been replaced by others which are still largely untouched. We are no longer so likely to suffer an early death from tuberculosis, gangrene or obstructed labour, but such improvements have been counterbalanced by newly dominant causes of morbidity and mortality, like lung cancer, heart disease, food poisoning and, most recently, AIDS. Many of the new afflictions are to some extent caused by the very same technological progress and changes in life-style which have led to the containment of the old. Examples are the toll exacted by road accidents (now the greatest single cause of death in male British teenagers), cancer due to the widespread prevalence of tobacco smoke and many other environmental carcinogens, heart disease encouraged by physical inactivity and an unhealthy diet of convenience, processed foods combined with the stress of modern phenomena such as mass unemployment and frustrating traffic jams, and sexually transmitted diseases spread more readily by an explosive increase in foreign and domestic travel and a more relaxed moral climate.

The reform of the abortion law in 1967 added a whole new dimension to British medicine. Nearly 170,000 legal abortions were carried out in 1988, which means that nearly 500 times each day doctors were 'servicing' rather than 'treating' their customers. Some members of the profession resent this role. The late Ian Donald, when Regius Professor of Midwifery at the University of Glasgow, once said to me, 'Well, you see, I'm a doctor. And therefore I will only do the operation [abortion] for doctors' reasons. I'm blowed if I'm just going to have something [sic] sent up to me with a note saying "Just get rid of this – it's inconvenient".'

Even the healers have contributed to the catalogue of new diseases and 'medical conditions' by introducing a whole range of illnesses caused by their attempts to heal – the so-called iatrogenic disorders (which can include death). An estimated 10 per cent of hospital admissions are people made sick by treatment instituted for some other complaint.

On the other hand, there have been dramatic improvements in certain health indices, like infant mortality and life expectancy at birth (as opposed to longevity). A hundred years ago a new-born boy could expect to survive to the age of forty-one, and a girl to the age of forty-five. These low average figures were due to the large numbers of deaths occurring among children and young adults, and especially to deaths during the first year of life. Only six out of every ten children born survived to adulthood, and the infant mortality rate (which is the number out of every 1,000 babies born alive dying before their first birthday) hovered around the 150 mark. By 1989 the figure for such deaths had fallen to just over eight per 1,000, of which the great majority occur within the first week of life – that is to say, among infants who are born less than fighting fit, because of prematurity, or as a result of a difficult labour, or because of some congenital abnormality, or, rarely, because of an acquired infection or inadequate care. (This does not apply to the Third World, where infection and malnutrition are the commonest causes of infant deaths.) As a result of the greatly reduced death rate among children and young people life expectancy at birth is now around seventy-two for men and seventy-seven for women.

However, this kind of 'success' simply creates new problems. Britain already contains almost a million people over the age of eighty-five, and that figure is likely to rise to 2 million by the middle of the next century, so doctors will become increasingly concerned with the time-consuming servicing of the old-aged. A recent estimate suggests that care for the over seventy-fives costs more than seven times the £200-odd per year now spent on health care and social services for citizens aged between sixteen and sixty-four.

The greatly improved chances of surviving for the *Book of Common Prayer*'s allowance of three-score years and ten (you see, things haven't changed a lot since 1662) have, infant mortality apart, been largely the result of a reduction in the toll exacted by infectious diseases. Since Gladstone first became prime minister, deaths from tuberculosis, typhoid, diphtheria, scarlet fever, whooping cough and measles have fallen by 99 per cent. Some of this improvement has been due to such factors as the widespread use of preventive inoculations, mass-radiography (for the early detection and treatment of tuberculosis before the victim could spread the disease), the development of penicillin and other anti-bacterial drugs, and similar instruments of medical science. But the trend was under way long before such weapons became available. Our infant mortality rate, for example, had fallen to around fifty by the outbreak of World War II, when the therapeutic revolution had hardly begun, and the assumption must be that the major force for change has been a better standard of living.

Marks and Spencer, offering excellent clothing at prices related to the national average wage, successive governments enabling local authorities to build sound houses for rent or purchase at prices also related to the national average wage, and companies like Sainsbury and the Co-Op and other providers of modestly priced foods for city dwellers, have probably, between them, had a larger impact on the health of the nation than all the medicines yet made. (Although they have also made it easier for the poor or ill-informed to subsist on filling, calorie-rich, but nutritionally inadequate 'junk foods'.)

Dr John Marks says that 'If all doctors stopped working tomorrow, and all we had instead was good water, clean air, and reasonable housing and food for everybody, that would do more for the population's health than we doctors do in all our lifetime.' That is a considerable statement, coming, as it did, from the then Chairman of the Council of the British Medical Association, who might be expected to promote the idea that his profession can claim the major credit for improvements in the nation's vital statistics.

WHO recognizes the limitations of the medical contribution to universal welfare, and says that 'Health for all requires the coordinated action of all sectors concerned. The health authorities can only deal with a part of the problem to be solved.' In his report on the Organization's work for 1988–9 the Director-General, Dr Hiroshi Nakajima, stressed that the health issues of the 1990s 'are inextricably related to issues of development and social equity'.

So what do doctors do? And what should they be trying to do?

Doctors have a vested interest in disease, and until quite recently were almost exclusively concerned with sickness, and hardly at all with health.

The medical texts I had to absorb as a student half a century ago concentrated largely on diagnosis. If a physician (less so in the case of a surgeon) could make a correct diagnosis, he had more or less done his job. Treatment was a secondary consideration because, of course, so few effective treatments were available, and the paragraphs on therapy were padded out with platitudes such as 'Pay attention to the bowels' or 'If it would not be an insult, advise a pregnant woman to take a bath daily'.

4

As a result of the paucity of worthwhile remedies the 'bedside manner' was a major weapon in the physician's armamentarium. He could often help most by instilling confidence and hope, and by sharing the burden of sickness with his patients and their relatives. Somebody who 'knew the answers' was in charge. The best doctors were as much priests as scientists.

The therapeutic revolution has changed all that. The modern attitude is that 'there is a pill for every ill', or, if there isn't, then there bloody well *ought* to be, and many doctors feel it is their duty to do something active in the face of every medical complaint. Patients in GPs' surgeries *have* to be sent out clutching a scrip for some drug which will 'solve' their problem, or, as Malcolm Muggeridge once put the matter, 'I will lift up mine eyes unto the pills, whence cometh my help.'

There is thus an epidemic of unnecessary, inappropriate and often harmful treatments, and not just with drugs. Heroic surgical procedures like heart and liver transplants top the catalogue of 'the miracles of modern medicine' although their impact on the health of the nation is negligible. The death of a patient is regarded as a lost game in the great professional tournament, so that cruel efforts are made to prolong lives which have clearly run their natural course.

The explosive growth of hi-tech, scientific medicine has seen a parallel diminution in the doctor's priestly role, partly, perhaps, because it is no longer regarded as an invaluable means of helping people cope with disease, compared, say, with the supposedly sure-fire effectiveness of a tranquillizer, and partly because the sheer manipulation and application of the plethora of remedies now available leaves little time for a softer, more human approach.

But, demonstrably, a significant proportion of human ills still cannot be assuaged by modern medical techniques. Moreover there is a growing popular unease concerning the impact of science and technology on the planet and its inhabitants. The pharmaceutical trade, which has created and supplies the great bulk of treatments offered by doctors, is an archetypal science-based industry. It is thus a favourite target for the darts of citizens who mistrust the hi-tech or 'unnatural' approach to life's problems, and who believe big business will go to any lengths in pursuit of profits, with small regard for the best interests of its customers. Family doctors, in particular, are sometimes regarded as little better than the retail end of the drug-makers' booming enterprise.

These factors may lie, in part at least, behind the remarkable growth of interest in alternative medicine, or 'dissident doctoring', whose practitioners are commonly happy to promise their clients relief from every kind of physical and mental ill. Indeed, an increasing sprinkling of 'proper' doctors now employ alternative approaches such as homoeopathy and acupuncture, while still freely using modern tools like penicillin and beta-blockers, but seeing in the former a means for offering help that they have found, frustratingly, they have not been able to provide from the orthodox armamentarium.

Writing in the *Journal of the Royal College of General Practitioners* in December 1989, Dr Jeremy Swayne, a Bristol consultant in homoeopathic medicine, claimed that 'there are three-quarters of a million consultations a year by doctors in the UK yielding homoeopathic prescriptions', sometimes because the doctors involved felt 'anxiety about the hazards of conventional medicine' and often because they wished to 'increase the scope of their therapeutic repertoire'.

Now, by and large alternative therapies are a load of simplistic, irrational, and mystical old rubbish. Homoeopathic theory, for example, is nonsensical to the scientific mind. Doctors who espouse the cult are therefore disregarding everything they were taught at medical school, where disease, diagnosis and treatment are presented as problems to be tackled by the logical application of tested and established knowledge. So why do they defect?

Perhaps because, after some experience on the job, they sense or recognize that the coldly 'clinical' approach falls sadly short of providing their clients with the kind of support and comfort they desire. Perhaps because their training failed to equip them for the task of practising medicine as an art as well as a science. So, lacking guidance from their tutors on the art of medicine, they look for help from gurus outside the ranks of the medical Establishment.

Samuel Hahnemann, the eighteenth-century Saxony physician who dreamt up homoeopathy, may have had some insupportable ideas, but he was well ahead of his time in preaching two important truths which have only recently won general respect. He insisted on

6

the need to treat the whole person and not just the disease (thus his choice of remedy would partly depend upon whether the patient was fat or thin, merry or morose), and he recognized that any medicine capable of doing good must also be capable of doing harm.

Latter-day medically qualified followers of Hahnemann are expressing, in a naive fashion, their discontent with the manner in which they are expected to perform. And the fact is that the customers of unorthodox practitioners often benefit greatly from 'irrational' treatments. This is because, lacking physically effective tools (just like the 'proper' doctors of half a century ago), the dissidents still make maximum use of sympathy and empathy and suggestion and persuasion. They spend time with their patients. They talk to them. They support them. They befriend them. They often offer them a good deal of common-sense, practical advice about how to cope with personal problems. They are the latter-day medical priests.

There will be a great need for curative medicine for very many years to come, and perhaps for so long as the race survives, but if doctors are to make their fullest possible contribution toward the ideal of 'Health for All by the Year 2000' (or whenever) they will have to discover how best to manipulate, in the words of Zanussi, 'the appliance of science'. In particular they will have to apply a far greater proportion of their energies and skills to the task of 'nursing' individuals and families, and even whole communities, and to preventing rather than curing disease, for it is crazy and, eventually, self-defeating, to devote the bulk of the resources available for health care to costly and often inefficient efforts designed to correct or ameliorate faults of the flesh which need never have happened in the first place.

Preventive medicine involves far more than broadening and intensifying the screening of citizens for the earliest manifestations of disease, or a vulnerability to disease, so that treatment can be instituted when it stands the best chance of achieving a cure or damage limitation. Indeed, this kind of exercise is not true prevention at all, but merely an extension of the curative approach.

True prevention involves a great deal of social engineering, which can only be achieved by politicians, but it also involves 'person engineering', which politicians cannot attempt.

Doctors occupy a position in society which allows them to influence, or attempt to influence, both politicians and individuals. But their current training ill fits them to the task of changing social and individual behaviour in a manner which will reduce the incidence of disease.

All medical students receive their clinical training in large general hospitals wherein the attitude towards the problems of sickness and health is fashioned by the consultants. But these are highly specialized experts who have achieved their influential posts by, in the words of the old saw, knowing more and more about less and less. Thus the most important formative years of medical neophytes are spent under the tutelage of powerful personalities who are marvellously knowledgeable concerning the functions and dysfunctions of the womb, but who may know damn all about women, or who may be dab hands at diagnosing and attempting to treat lung cancer, but who haven't a clue about why people smoke.

It is true that all medical schools now strive to teach their pupils a little bit about general practice, and may even own a professor in the subject. And it is true that after graduation, and at least another year in junior hospital posts, young physicians have to serve an apprenticeship in family doctoring before becoming employable by the NHS as principals in the trade. But this additional training is largely aimed at giving the new GP some familiarity with the kind of medical problems not seen in hospital practice (some 90 per cent of all incidents of illness are dealt with by GPs without referral to specialists), and with the organizational aspects of primary health care. It does little to modify the hospital-bred belief that the chief purpose of medicine is the management of established disease.

The nature of the courses offered by most of the London medical colleges (where one-third of British doctors are trained) further favours the production of graduates with a blinkered view of the real world. Students undergo an intensive two years of pre-clinical instruction (mainly in anatomy, physiology and biochemistry) in schools which are physically part of a teaching hospital complex and divorced from the rest of the university. Thus most doctors qualify in their early twenties, having been largely isolated, since the age of eighteen, from their contemporaries who are studying other subjects or doing different jobs. They know very little about the skills and

8

attitudes and interests and aspirations of other kinds of worker in the health and welfare business (nurses, social workers, pharmacists, health visitors, and so on), let alone those of their fellow citizens who have nothing to do with the medical trade.

Only one of my respondents thought the current medical curriculum adequate. The rest thought it more or less appalling. Why hasn't it changed? For the same reason, I suppose, that a supertanker in the English Channel is quite incapable of changing course when it's still a couple of miles away from a foreseen disaster. Behemoths suffer from inertia.

So perhaps both a drastic revision of the manner in which doctors are educated and an equally revolutionary change in the manner in which they operate will have to come about before the medical profession can contribute effectively to the task of achieving 'Health for All by the Year 2000' (or whenever).

2   *What Are Doctors For?*

Injury and disease have been common elements in the experience of living organisms since life began, and earliest Man must have sought ways to assuage suffering.

It's a fair guess that there have been individuals who had, or who pretended to, special skills in the art of healing ever since our species began to live in groups, and such commonly self-appointed gurus would have been patronized by other members of the tribe, because it is a characteristic of our race that we love to believe in 'experts' – from heads of state to agony aunts – who, we assume, must somehow know how to save us from the consequences of our foolish ways.

So healers were probably marked-out members of society from the start, and they were (and frequently still are) often also priests (or whatever the local equivalent might be), because of a popular view that illness is God-given, or the malign work of other spiritual or magical forces, or that, even if it isn't, those same forces can, if they will, suspend the workings of natural laws and intervene on the sufferer's behalf. Thus it made sense for invalids to seek the help of those among their fellows who were supposed to have a hot line to the other world.

Explain it how you will, doctors, in one guise or another, have been around since Man began, and they stand apart in the ranks of the professions for one very good reason.

Parsons and lawyers (not to mention accountants, teachers, bankers, journalists, soldiers, politicians, and all the other ragtags and bobtails who now like to call themselves 'professionals') deal with man-made ideas and institutions and situations, and the human race could very well survive without them.

Healers, by contrast, deal with problems innate to Man's biological make-up and his place in the natural world, and the need for medicine (if not necessarily doctors) is for ever.

But what are doctors for today?

Some of my respondents found no need to hesitate before answering this 64,000-dollar question. The doctor's job is to relieve suffering by curing, or, if that is not possible, by attempting to alleviate ills of the body and the mind. It's as simple as that. The easy-answerers then usually demonstrated their awareness of the currently fashionable mood by hastily adding that the profession must also be equally or even more concerned to prevent disease happening in the first place by paying ever more attention to such interventions as screenings and inoculations, and, above all, its members must devote ample time to counselling, in an effort to persuade their clients to lead less disease-inviting lives.

Certainly one of the primary functions expected of doctors is the relief of suffering. What does that involve?

One fairly good answer to the question was given by Dr Francis Dudley Hart, an Honorary Consultant Physician to the Westminster Hospital in London, when he addressed a symposium on 'People as Patients and Patients as People', organized by the Office of Health Economics in 1988.

Dr Hart is a rheumatologist. He deals with patients who often suffer gross disability and intractable pain because of arthritis, and who may be anxious and depressed because of their condition. He has to decide how to assess and how to prescribe for and how to advise such unfortunates.

He said that a doctor in his specialty 'has to be an able diagnostician, applied pharmacologist, rehabilitation expert and physiotherapist, psychiatrist, and sometimes a kind of father confessor, and always a sympathetic human being'.

Dr Hart's analysis of the role of the rheumatologist could well be applied to any doctor faced by any client, but, while it reveals his profession's conceit that doctors must bear the responsibility for every aspect of a patient's needs, it lacks mention of other essential functions which today's medical journeyman is expected to embrace.

Professor Nicholas Bosanquet, from the viewpoint of a sociologist, sees the relief of pain and suffering and the provision of reassurance as an essential but in some respects secondary part of the medical mission, and emphasizes the importance of first achieving an effective system for delivering medical care, both at a personal and a social level, for the business of treating patients is undertaken within a framework of programmes and by the use of resources whose nature or allocation have already been determined.

Getting the system right involves a managerial approach and the mobilization of teams of workers possessed of a wide variety of different skills. Doctors, Professor Bosanquet suggests, have largely excluded themselves from this process. As a result of the stereotyped nature of medical education, coupled with a lack of leadership from the top, they have allowed themselves to become isolated on one side of the health system, and other people have been coming in to make the key decisions. He regards this as a lost opportunity, and believes that in a sense doctors are becoming increasingly under-used in relation to their academic background and ability and potential.

One cause of this diminution of the medical influence in medical affairs may be the fact that for some time now medical school places have been increasingly filled from the ranks of academic high-flyers of a kind Professor Bosanquet labels 'approved adolescents'. These are young people who have 'done all the right things'. They are 'white males and white females from the suburbs'. He has nothing against such paragons, but claims that they do not, on the whole, develop the kind of leadership and entrepreneurial drive needed to get things done in society. The people who do stir things up have usually been 'unapproved adolescents – the ones who've had to live with the disapproval of peer groups and superiors, and who tend to be bolder at innovating'. But it has become more and more difficult for unapproved adolescents to get into medical school. 'So,' Professor Bosanquet says, 'medicine, for one reason or another, has cut itself off from a world in which there's more change and more flexibility and more innovation and more of an enterprise culture.'

This reduction of the control which doctors now exert over the manner in which they function may account for the findings of a recent survey which suggested that very nearly half of all medical graduates of five years' standing wished that they had not gone into medicine. Professor Bosanquet believes that a sense of this lack of job satisfaction (whatever its cause) has filtered down to school-leavers, so that, over the course of the next ten or fifteen years a smaller proportion of young people will want to commit themselves to the medical life. But he comments that this may have the good effect of forcing medical schools to accept a wider range of applicants, with a consequent enrichment of the ranks.

It used to be a central article of the medical faith that a doctor's prime duty was to do the very best he could for each individual patient. It was a one-to-one contract, and nobody else's interests were involved. But, as Professor George Teeling Smith, speaking as an economist, somewhat brutally put it, 'Doctors have to realize that the nature of their responsibility has changed dramatically since the 1930s when there was very little they could do for patients anyway, so it didn't matter if they wasted their resources. We now have a very different situation where you have a housebound patient down the road who needs a new hip and who needs a quarter-of-an-hour of your time twice a week, but doesn't get it because you're wasting that time chatting up a hypochondriac and wasting a resource, time being the most valuable resource of any profession, and it should be used for those most able to benefit from it.'

He is making the point that one of the major responsibilities of the modern doctor is the wise rationing of health care, because the demand is infinite and the supply is not.

Health care for the benefit of the individual (as opposed to public health measures, such as confining diphtheria victims or lunatics, or the universal vaccination of infants against smallpox) has in fact always been rationed. In pre-NHS times the cost to the patient was the regulating factor. The poor (apart from the limited service provided for workers under the old panel system) often simply could not afford skilled attention, and unless they developed some 'interesting' condition, which qualified them for admission to one of the voluntary or municipal hospitals (always supposing such an institution to be within their physical reach), they largely had to fend for themselves. Certainly doctors were not much concerned to parcel out their services in a manner best calculated to benefit the common weal. They dealt with the sick who came their way and the rest were ignored.

With the advent of free medical care for all at the time of need the situation changed completely, and doctors, perforce, became managers, or at least dispensers, of vast new resources funded from the public purse, and in so far as they failed to accept this new managerial role, or to prove effective in it, they laid themselves open to becoming ever more managed themselves.

The original myth, believed by politicians if not by the more far-sighted members of the medical profession, was that the national health would so improve under the new arrangements that the demand would be self-limiting and costs would eventually actually fall.

The opposite has happened. More and more conditions have become treatable, more and more citizens are surviving to suffer the many ailments of old age, and more and more elaborate and expensive therapies have become available, so that, although the NHS has become the country's largest industry and employer, and although the service cost the taxpayer some £26 billion in 1989, the gap between demand and supply has become ever larger and more obvious.

Thus an effort to relate the use of resources, both human and material and financial, to the benefits they produce, has become an essential and urgent part of the task of keeping the ship afloat. It is this central task, with all the implications it has for the manner in which doctors are able to operate on a day-to-day and person-to-person basis, which the medical profession has largely allowed to fall into the hands of 'outsiders'.

The new contracts for general practitioners, involving cash limits for prescribing and offering GPs the chance (which could become the requirement) to accept budgets from which to purchase hospital and other services for their patients, and the move to allow hospitals to become self-governing and not only to sell their services within the system but to choose what kind of services to offer, are harsh examples of the manner in which outsiders (in this case our present Government) are attempting to force doctors to become managers.

But is that really what doctors are for? Is Professor Bosanquet right in claiming that the profession has missed out on the chance to play the major role in controlling its own destiny and the shape of the medical services within which it operates?

What are doctors for?

Dr Raanan Gillon, who is both a working physician and a

graduate philosopher, and a powerful force in the realm of medical ethics, states, simply, that doctors are for helping people. 'That's quite important,' he says. 'Students are told not to say at their admission interview that "I want to help people" because that's supposed to turn the interviewers off.

'It's a load of old rubbish. Of course that's why most people want to go into medicine, and I believe that's now becoming an acceptable reason again. All this stiff upper lip business about an enthusiasm for medical science, or improving the health of the nation, or whatever, is giving way to the original intention.

'It's worth reiterating that the primary task is helping people who are ill rather than people who are well. It's an important distinction to make in the face of the current emphasis on prevention and the claim that to prevent is vastly better than to cure.

'There's a real conceptual problem here which people fail to recognize, because it doesn't matter how much prevention you undertake, you'll always have illness at the end of it – either the same illness that you've merely delayed rather than prevented, or another illness which replaces the one you *have* prevented. There'll still be people who are ill and dying, and medicine's primary function is to help the ill and dying – to try and ameliorate their nasty symptoms, and to help them not to die if they don't want to die, and, of course, not to prevent them from dying when they do.

'I'm actually very worried about equating prevention and health promotion with looking after ill people because with a fixed budget and limited resources, the more you do for the healthy the less you can do for the ill.'

I asked Dr Gillon whether a significant shift of resources towards preventive medicine might not so reduce illness that doctors would still have ample time to serve all the needs of the sick as well.

'That seems to me to be a real myth – one that Beveridge himself believed. All that would happen is that you'd delay illness. Occasionally you can come out with a preventive mechanism which is actually efficient to the extent that it stops a particular problem. But we're mortal beings and will go on being mortal beings for the foreseeable future.'

Dr Gillon agrees that a great deal remains to be done in the matter of trying to prevent preventable diseases, and that this is a highly desirable activity, but that it is wrong, for example, to equate political moves aimed at stopping people smoking with the treatment of smokers who have contracted lung cancer, and to regard the first as being equally or even more desirable than the second because it produces more hedons. They are, he says, two different enterprises.

So is the traditional role of the doctor – to help the individual sick person – still the right one, and should the profession be content to concentrate on this prime function, and to leave the many other important aspects of health care to others?

One response to this question would be to point out that there is a wide range of quite different kinds of doctor, and that it is unrealistic to lump them all together and then ask, 'What is a doctor for?' The Chief Medical Officer to the Department of Health, and a medical man on the board of a pharmaceutical company, and a pathologist in an institute for medical research, may never set eyes on a sick person in a professional mode from one year's end to another, yet all can contribute importantly to health care.

Professor Bosanquet regrets that doctors have not sufficiently espoused the managerial role. Dr Gillon is worried that they may be diluting their prime function by engaging in activities which are not their true concern. Who is right?

I suspect that Gillon comes nearer to the truth, to the extent that most kinds of doctor should concentrate on helping people – one to one. They should be content as members, and not necessarily always the leaders, of health care teams, and should not assume that they, and they alone, have a God-given right to deal with, or at any rate control, all health affairs. There are many others who are better qualified and better placed to deal with many of the obstacles in the way of achieving 'Health for All by the Year 2000' (or whenever).

The Role of Nurses

Nurses, if only by reason of their numbers (there are some half million on the 'active' list in the UK), are perhaps the most obvious of the non-medically qualified professionals who share responsibility for health care with the medical profession, but they feel undervalued. As a senior nurse administrator once put it to me,

'Nursing is perceived as "women's work", and it's widely believed that you don't need to be educated to be a nurse.' That this perception of nurses is shared by many doctors is confirmed by conversations I've had with graduate and undergraduate nurses, who have found that their relationship with doctors becomes much easier once their academic status is made known. The doctors suddenly start talking to them as though they were intelligent fellow professionals. The fact that the doctors had not been doing so before is a pretty good indication of their opinion of the 'ordinary' member of the tribe's intellectual capacity and position in the scheme of things.

A typical attitude was voiced by Ellis Downes, who was in the middle of his first postgraduate year of hospital jobs when I spoke to him. I had put it to him that there is a considerable lack of understanding between nurses and doctors concerning the nature of their respective roles.

'Yes, and the gap is growing. Nurses are taking less and less responsibility for patient care, and there's a growing sense of unease among junior doctors that they're being asked to undertake more and more trivial tasks because nurses don't want the responsibility – things like giving intravenous drugs. We don't spend five years at medical school just to learn how to inject a drug into someone. Nurses simply don't want to know. They won't, for example, take an intravenous tube out of a patient now. A doctor's got to do it. They want to keep their noses clean.

'The moment anything goes wrong they're on the phone. "Just to let you know that Mrs Bloggs' temperature's gone up to 38°." Then they write on the nursing card "Mrs Bloggs' T noted to be 38° – Dr Downes informed" – abnegating all responsibility.

'It's a growing trend, and we junior doctors are getting fed up with it. There are a few good nurses who perform fantastically, but on the whole they're willing to take less and less responsibility. They're happy just to make beds and give out the occasional drug.'

A very different view is taken by Dr James Malone-Lee, a young consultant geriatrician on the staff of University College Hospital, London. Dr Malone-Lee (unlike Professor Bosanquet) believes that the NHS 'has been far too dominated by the doctors, who are far too powerful in their control over what happens', and he has successfully and profitably given the nurses working in his department (and also his patients) much more responsibility for the way in which things are done.

'Nurses can be encouraged to voice their discontent about the way you, as a doctor, handle patients. It's all kept tight inside them, because they're taught not to challenge too much, but, given the chance, it will all come out.

'They are very sensitive to you rushing, and not making things clear, and not giving patients the time and the opportunity to say what they wanted to say.

'There's also considerable emphasis on having you explain why you want to use such and such a drug – what are the good reasons for doing so? This can be quite fatiguing, but it also produces quite good prescribing habits, because if you know when writing a prescription that you may have to justify it in quite some depth to a nurse who's going to question you, then you're much more careful.

'In this department nurses were asked to be punctilious about asking why we were doing things if they had any doubts. We expect them to lecture to others, because we have quite a big training programme here, and if they're not clear on why things are done, they'd soon get found out when teaching.

'I know that nurses in one of the country's leading departments of geriatrics, which is held up as a model, and is run by a most energetic doctor, are very unhappy because the place is dominated by the medical juggernaut which gives them no opportunity to express their views. The doctors think they're the great experts, but the nurses' view tells a different story.

'There are some areas of medicine where the nurses' role is quite limited, as, for example, in acute surgery. The patients come in and have their operation and forty-eight hours later they're better, and on their way, and don't really require much nursing care. It's all in the realm of the surgeons who know what they're up to, and that's fine. But there are other areas where the overlap between what the doctors are doing and what the nurses are doing is very considerable, and in geriatrics in particular the overlap is huge.

'It's important that doctors and nurses think hard about this, so that doctors move away from some areas in which they now have a powerful influence to others in which they can use their skills to better advantage. There's no point, for example, in doctors doing interminable rounds in rehabilitation wards offering advice and instructions to the specialist workers. It's crazy for me to think I can tell a physiotherapist or an occupational therapist how to rehabilitate someone.

'And you allow the nurses to judge when patients need the attention of a doctor and when they don't. They're qualified to do that. Outside hospital people decide for themselves when they want to see a doctor. Inside you can leave it to the nurses. No problem.

'I act as the equivalent of a houseman to my long-stay and rehabilitation wards, and they call me when they want me. They telephone me perhaps once a day and I go up and do what I'm told. And I find that the medicine I practise there is infinitely more difficult than it used to be because I'm presented with problems which the nurses have thought about, and they've only asked me there because they do have a complex problem.

'Working in this way has made the life-style on these wards so much better, which is reflected in the fact that the nurses are staying, and we don't have a recruitment problem. They only leave for promotion or to have a baby.

'But when you advocate this kind of approach doctors panic, and think they'll be left with nothing to do. That's rubbish. We've been using the rituals of ward rounds and providing unwelcome advice in various sectors as an excuse for not getting stuck into problems which *should* be attracting our attention.'

Dr Malone-Lee is convinced that his approach could be well employed in the acute medical sector, and not just in the care of the old ill where the nursing is self-evidently of prime importance.

'When I was doing general medicine my effective input took place within the first twenty-four to forty-eight hours, and then the patients were mostly getting better, and after that I was just being meddlesome and a damned nuisance to everybody. It would have been much better to withdraw and let the nurses get on with their side of the job. But to do that you have to retreat from some of the traditional approaches – the 'ward round' in particular, and especially the 'retinue' ward round, which is a very discourteous way of approaching patients, and also wholly inappropriate to the care of the vast majority.

'But it still goes on. It's claimed that if you abandoned it you'd lose out on teaching. I don't believe that at all. If you don't have a retinue you end up teaching far more people far more effectively. I can see no justification for it at all, and it must be removed if you're going to allow nurses and other people the room they need to do their jobs.'

When Dr Malone-Lee first started airing his ideas he met a lot of opposition, with colleagues thinking them anathema and him a maverick, but more recently he has found growing sympathy and interest. Certainly many doctors are now at least paying lip-service to the view that nurses cover some important aspects of health care better than they can themselves, and that nurses should be regarded as professionals in their own right, and not merely as handmaidens to the medical profession.

David Owen goes so far as to claim that the still unsatisfactory status of nurses constitutes the biggest problem currently facing the NHS. They are leaving the profession in droves. There must, says Dr Owen, be a dramatic improvement in incentives to stay in, with better conditions and hours of work. There must be facilities like crèches and car parks (no longer to be considered a luxury reserved for consultants), and nurses must be used for more responsible tasks, which could certainly include prescribing. There must be a continuing reduction in the number of housekeeping and other non-nursing jobs now loaded on to nurses' shoulders.

Dr Derek Cracknell, a senior GP and Chairman of the Cambridgeshire Family Practitioner Committee (FPCs, further described in Chapter 5, are now called Family Health Services Authorities), is a strong advocate of the practice team, because he, too, does not believe that 'doctors know everything best, and we never have done, and if we're honest with ourselves we know that's so. In many cases a homely nurse can provide a young mother, away from grandma and her own mum, with a much better service than I can. A pat on the shoulder at the right time is of great benefit.'

But it is by no means just a question of the occasional need for a softer and less dauntingly clinical approach than doctors commonly adopt. A good practice team, says Dr Cracknell, should consist of people possessing a variety of skills, with the patient able to make a rational choice about the type of help to seek. Ideally, if a practice is to operate a comprehensive programme of primary health care, the team should include not just doctors and nurses, but other professionals such as a chiropodist and a physiotherapist and, perhaps most importantly, a counsellor able to advise on a whole range of personal problems from a rocky marriage to dealing with the social services. And a practice manager, in addition to the more usual receptionists, can greatly increase efficiency and leave the members of the medical team with more time to do their proper jobs. But while Dr Cracknell fully appreciates the value of the practice nurse, he admits that 'We don't like people poaching from us, so we've tended to keep them but give them menial jobs.'

Pharmacists' Skills Ignored

Britain's 36,000 pharmacists feel undervalued and under-used – at least the three-quarters of them who end up running High Street chemists' shops do. Pharmacists undergo a training not much less onerous, and certainly requiring no less academic ability and application for its successful completion, than that imposed on medical students. In the old days the dispensing chemist actually made up pills and potions according to the elaborate recipes scribbled by doctors, and for this task special knowledge and skills were essential. But nowadays virtually all the High Street chemist has to do in order to fulfil his contract with the NHS is hand out the correct amounts of the ready-made products of the pharmaceutical industry. His considerable learning is totally wasted on this mundane and mechanical task. He does have a duty to check on the accuracy of prescriptions (about 5 per cent of those presented to dispensaries contain some error or omission which has to be queried), and he can land himself in serious trouble, up to and including a criminal charge, if a patient should suffer or, as has happened, die, because of a failure to exercise this care. He may spot the fact that a customer is taking an incompatible or even dangerous mixture of drugs. This is a valuable and occasionally a life-saving function, but a computer on the doctor's consulting room desk could do the job as well, and the High Street chemist may be a dying breed.

However, pharmacists do have an expert knowledge of aspects of drugs and drug usage of a kind not commonly possessed by doctors (as well as a good grounding in human biology), and they feel that the quality of prescribing could be greatly improved if they were involved at the outset in the planning of treatment, such as considering the best way of administering a particular remedy. This does happen in some hospitals, where, in addition, a pharmacist may interview patients on admission to establish their medication history (whether they have had adverse drug reactions in the past, whether they are currently taking drugs prescribed elsewhere or bought over the counter, and so on). He may also monitor (as by the assay of drugs in body fluids) how patients' bodies are handling medicines taken while in hospital, and counsel patients on how to use the medicines they may have to take after discharge, and the possible side-effects to look out for. Doctors are frequently neglectful of such matters, even if they carry in their heads the necessary knowledge.

One medical unit experienced a ten-fold increase in the recognition and reporting of adverse drug reactions after adding a pharmacist to the clinical team and found that, roughly twice a day, the pharmacist had been able to offer advice leading to a significant improvement in the treatment schedules which the doctors had originally proposed.

This is a prime example of the manner in which a humble acceptance of the superficially threatening proposition that the doctor doesn't necessarily always know best can lead to a better service to the customer (which is what the whole thing ought to be about). It is also an illustration of the waste of talent and human resources which occurs when the medical profession insists on its monopoly of wisdom.

Covering

'Covering' has long been one of the cardinal sins on the medical calendar, which, in the past, has cost many a doctor his place on the Medical Register. The term is used to describe a situation where a doctor is in cahoots with some non-medical person in a fashion that allows that person to treat patients or provide some other medical service under the umbrella of the covering doctor's professional status and qualifications.

The stated purpose of the prohibition of this practice was the protection of the public against the ministrations of unskilled charlatans, but in reality the profession's strong antipathy to covering stemmed from a determination to protect its profitable monopoly of the healing trade, and the fear of being accused of covering persists.

Thus Sir Robert Kilpatrick, President of the General Medical Council, clinical pharmacologist and enlightened educational reformist, told me that his Council had recently been asked whether it was acceptable for a non-medical person to perform an operation under a surgeon's supervision. The query related to a proposal from Oxford, now implemented, that a specially trained nurse should remove from a patient's leg the sections of vein required by the surgeon for a coronary by-pass operation. It is a purely technical procedure, but, as Sir Robert pointed out, it raises the question of whether nurses or operating theatre technicians or whoever could be entrusted with a wide range of surgical interventions which are purely technical in kind, and how far the devolution of medical responsibility should go.

What distinguishes the doctor from the nurse or technician to the extent that, in Sir Robert's view, many tasks should always be reserved to his profession?

'The specific difference is that in his training he learns about aetiology. He goes through the discipline of causation, which is not done in that kind of detail in the training of any other members of the caring team, and so much flows from that.' The surgeon, says Sir Robert, knows a great deal about surgical pathology, but clearly could not understand aetiology and pathology without a thorough appreciation of normal structure and function – a knowledge of physiology, anatomy and histology (which is just micro-anatomy), and of biochemistry.

'There's this one nurse doing vein dissections in Oxford, but I can't imagine we'd ever get to the position when we say, "This individual needs the gall bladder removed, and it's a technical procedure, so we'll hand it over to a surgical technician," because that technician could open up the abdomen and find something he doesn't understand. There's a lump, or there's an unusual appearance of the gut, and to know how to proceed he needs an understanding of aetiology.

'A classic example would be that of a patient who's referred because he's vomiting. If you take the technical approach you'd say, "He's vomiting, therefore send him to somebody who's an expert on the stomach." But he may be vomiting because of increased intracranial pressure, and you need somebody who appreciates that possibility, and who'll examine his eyes for possible signs of such a cause – somebody versed in aetiology.'

Few would wish to deny that many medical activities ought to remain the prerogative of doctors, not for the benefit of the profession, but for the sake of the consumer. I wouldn't want a district nurse or health visitor (or even my friendly neighbourhood GP, for that matter) to undertake sole responsibility for my care if I happened to be unfortunate enough to fall victim to leukaemia. On the other hand, if I developed senile diabetes then I'd quite possibly be better off under the care of one of the new breed of nurses specializing in the care of patients with particular diseases (such as diabetes) than following the advice of my GP. And if I fell unconscious and pulseless from a heart attack in my village High Street I'd rather have the rapid attention of an ambulance crew trained in sophisticated resuscitation techniques, and equipped with oxygen and appropriate drugs and a defibrillator, than the charitable and more deeply informed (aetiologically speaking) help of a passing orthopaedic surgeon who'd probably have only a vague and ill-remembered and certainly under-rehearsed idea of how to save my life.

So even in the matter of dealing with the medical needs of an individual patient there can be circumstances under which a non-medical professional can perform as well as or even better than a fully licensed member of the healing guild.

With the explosive development of electronic aids which can give expert 'instructions' to their non-expert users, the list of such circumstances is bound to grow. But many doctors still tend to believe that they should be the final arbiters in every health-related issue.

In 1989 the BMA purchased full-page advertising space in the national press as part of the Association's propaganda against the Government's proposed NHS reforms. 'What do you call a person who doesn't accept medical advice?' they asked. Answer, 'Kenneth

Clarke' – the unfortunate if somewhat abrasive Health Minister involved. It was a silly stunt, which probably did little to recruit extra support from an electorate already unhappy about apparent threats to its strangely beloved health service. But it did most marvellously reveal the medical profession's conceit that the commonality will swallow the idea that doctors always know best, and that the profession's views should prevail, not only in the clinical realms of treatment and disease, but also in every other aspect of health care, from determining how available resources should be used to regulating what the *hoi polloi* may be permitted to eat and drink, and even including whether or not the so-called sport of boxing should be allowed.

Perhaps the medical profession is weakening itself by attempting to assume far too large a range of responsibilities, and is losing status and credibility because of an evident failure to succeed in ventures it should never have entertained. But it would be naive and simplistic in the extreme to insist that doctors should confine the use of their knowledge and skills to the task of helping the individual sick person. In today's society we will only succeed in managing things well if the many experts available (from plumbers to politicians) can manage to work as a team, sharing their understandings, and not just allowing but actively welcoming and using the cooperation of 'outsiders'. The 'closed shop' is a recipe for stagnation.

Dr Joe Collier, who is a clinical pharmacologist at St George's Hospital in London, and a noted medical iconoclast, stresses the role of doctors as researchers, with the task of feeding information into the system, and he, like Professor Bosanquet, is dismayed that so much of the current work on such matters as the pattern and causes of ill health and the appropriate deployment of resources is being done by outsiders such as non-medically trained sociologists and economists and epidemiologists. He thinks it ludicrous, for example, that almost all the research in the high-powered cardiac unit of his own hospital is done on treatment and almost none on prevention, holding that work of the latter kind should be undertaken by people 'deep inside medicine', because it is only doctors who carry any significant clout when it comes to lobbying the Establishment.

Is this a valid argument, or is it just a rationalization of a gut feeling that 'doctors know best'?

What are doctors for?

Clearly the testing of approaches to the treatment of, say, blocked coronary arteries *is* predominantly a medical (or clinical) exercise, even though other kinds of experts like biochemists and laser technologists may be crucially involved. But it was a physicist, Röntgen, who discovered x-rays. It was a chemist, Pasteur, who established the germ theory of disease, and another chemist, Domagk, who developed Prontosil, the first of the now wide range of rapidly effective and comparatively non-toxic anti-bacterial drugs. The monk and biologist, J. G. Mendel, with his rows of peas, laid the foundations of the science of heredity, and it was the biologist Watson and the physicist Crick who explained the mechanisms involved, and so sparked the explosive growth of molecular biology, with all its profound implications for the day-to-day management of disease. It was a physiologist, Robert Edwards, whose work led to the birth of Louise Joy Brown, the first test-tube baby, in 1978, and to all that has followed that event. The list of non-medical people whose researches have shaped the nature of modern medical practice is a long one, and, left to themselves, doctors would have achieved only a fraction of their present ability to 'help people'.

Of course, doctors, too, have been responsible for very many major advances in medical science, but it is salutary to recognize the fact that medicine, probably to a larger extent than any other profession, makes use of and is indebted to the efforts and insights of workers in other fields, and if this is acceptable in the realm of clinical practice, why should doctors not be equally willing to acknowledge the contributions to health care which can be made by all manner of men and women outside the guild?

This is not to suggest that doctors should concentrate solely on the work of the surgery and clinic and ward and operating theatre, and on research directly related to the problems to be tackled in such places, relinquishing all responsibility for wider or more peripheral issues to others. But if the profession were willing to loosen its grip on much of its perceived sphere of influence, and could subdue its antagonism to 'interference' from 'outsiders', it might find life a great deal easier and more rewarding. Perhaps almost half of recent graduates would not regret having chosen medicine as a career if the system freed them from many a burdensome and energy-consuming duty and chore, so that they could indeed spend their working hours in helping people.

3   *Doctors and Disease*

Most doctors are not particularly interested in health. By inclination and training they are devoted to the study of disease. It is sick, not healthy people, who crowd their surgeries and out-patient departments and fill their hospital beds, and it is the fact that the population can be relied upon to provide a steady flow of sufferers from faults of the mind and of the flesh that guarantees them a job and an income in harsh times as in fair.

It is true that 'preventive medicine' and 'health education' are currently buzz phrases in the medical world, but medical students have their professional attitudes formed in institutions which, apart from a few areas like midwifery, are almost exclusively devoted to dealing with people who are, to some degree, unwell or disabled, and who seek a cure. If, after graduation, the new doctor chooses a career in hospital medicine, he remains in a situation where his prime function is to 'do something' for every in-patient and out-patient in his charge. And if he goes into general practice he will largely be faced by customers who have come to his surgery or asked for a home visit because they expect 'something to be done' for a real or imaginary ill.

Today's doctor can, indeed, 'do something' useful in the way of active treatment for a considerable proportion of his clients, but there remain many situations where a little reassurance or advice may be the best and only medicine required. However, masterly inactivity is a difficult stance to assume. Patients find it hard to believe that there may not indeed be a suitable pill (or other remedy) for their particular ill, and doctors find it hard to admit to their patients (or even to themselves) that they can't always pull a curative rabbit out of their Aesculapian top hats.

A great deal of the modern doctor's attitude towards disease is shaped by the nature of his pharmacopoeia. General practitioners now have some 2,000 prescription medicines at their disposal, and rely predominantly on this resource when striving to meet their customers' needs, but have not been taught to ask themselves, 'What is my objective in using drugs?' and then to go on to ask, 'Have I achieved it?'

David Ryde, a South London family doctor, has gained a reputation for himself within the profession for his missionary zeal in preaching the virtue of moderation in the use of medicines. He has managed a successful practice for many years despite having reduced his prescribing levels to around 20 per cent of the national average. He once told a conference how he had recently issued only eleven prescriptions during the course of 100 consecutive consultations, and that this, for him, was a not uncommon achievement. He has pointed out that many reports have shown that in over half of the consultations taking place in general practice no clear diagnosis is made, but that, nevertheless, over 70 per cent of patients leave the surgery clutching a prescription. In other words, family doctors are frequently instructing their clients to swallow, sniff, dab on, or otherwise mix strange substances with their flesh, not because the prescriber has identified a specific bodily fault which the chosen chemical might, on scientific grounds, be calculated to assuage or correct, but simply to 'do something' by offering a remedy known or alleged to be 'effective' in the general realm of the customer's complaint, such as insomnia, or anxiety, or a pain in the belly after food, or a wheezy chest, and without determining why such symptoms are present.

'Most prescribing is unnecessary,' says Dr Ryde. 'What patients need is understanding and insight about whatever bugs them, rather than being fobbed off with a scrip. But it's so hard to get this across to most of them.'

He claims that most of his local colleagues say, 'Why put your head on the chopping block? Give them something.' But 'that's "medicalizing" the situation. You're confirming that your patient needs something in order to get better. Not only that, but you're maintaining an expectation, so that when you want to educate patients into how to stay healthy you can't, because you're encouraging them to think that they should only come to you when they think there's something wrong.'

When you prescribe for patients, Dr Ryde says, you're confirming that they're ill. 'They come in with one problem and go out with two.'

There is no doubt that many prescriptions are issued for a variety of wrong or inadequate reasons, perhaps the commonest being the fact that it's a convenient and traditional way to end a consultation. David Ryde recounts how he once discussed this problem with an elderly doctor who had been in practice for many years before the coming of the NHS. 'He told me that up until 1948 every patient was sent away with a bottle of medicine for which they paid 6d (that's six old pence). The bottle cost him 2d and the medicine cost him 2d leaving 2d profit. But he always got the patients to bring their bottles back, and he always diluted the medicine by half, so the whole lot cost him 1d, and he made 5d profit on every consultation. He couldn't suddenly abandon the routine with the arrival of the NHS. His patients had come to expect treatment. A visit to the doctor was equated with treatment. So he just had to carry on. He was hoist with his own petard, as I presume every other doctor in the country was as well.

'That coincided with the drug industry rearing its head, so instead of the patients getting mostly harmless coloured juleps they started getting active agents – perhaps only vitamins or iron – and although these might be regarded as placebos they *are* active drugs, and not entirely harmless, as we now know. Give patients iron just to fend them off and you may occasionally damage them.'

Drugs may also be inappropriately prescribed in an effort to forestall trouble before it has occurred, or to treat symptoms *before* a firm diagnosis has been made, or simply as an easy method of responding to a complex problem.

Derek Cracknell acknowledges these happenings, but suggests that the evils resulting from bad prescribing habits may have been overplayed. 'Perhaps we have relied too much on medication, and have tended to overuse two products – antibiotics and the psychotropics' (like penicillin and Valium).

He explains that this is particularly true in the case of certain diseases. When, for example, children are brought in with an upper respiratory tract infection and a sore throat they are frequently prescribed an antibiotic right away, despite the fact that such conditions are almost always caused by viruses, against which antibiotics are wholly ineffective. But it is an insurance against the fairly modest risk of a secondary bacterial infection in, say, the ear, developing later. 'So there's a great tendency to say, "Right – better to give them penicillin the first time round, whether they need it or not, because it's not going to do them a great deal of harm." And maybe not a great deal of good either, but at least you've prevented Mum bringing the child back two days later, saying, "He's not better yet."

'The same applies to psychotropics [drugs, like tranquillizers, which affect the mind]. Instead of taking on this great role as counsellor-cum-father-figure-cum-priest-cum-whatever, it's easier to say, "Right – if I give you this it will help you settle down more quickly. I've given you a prop to hold on to. This is your prop through life, to make life easier for you." And we felt good doing this. Doctors do feel good providing help. That's one of the reasons why we're in the profession.'

Dr Cracknell made several further pertinent remarks on this theme. 'We have used the drugs the pharmaceutical companies produce for us, and that has been recognized as a way of providing care. This has rebounded on us to some extent, but I don't think nearly as much as the scare stories suggest, otherwise we'd have a lot more people suing us and (lacking the free use of psychotropics by GPs) a lot more people in mental hospitals. . . . Doctors will change too readily to a new medicine hoping it will be the new panacea. That doesn't make them any different from Mrs Bloggs who thinks one washing powder will be better than another. Doctors are as gullible as other people, and if a rep comes round and tells us that this is the best thing since sliced bread we are likely to think that they've done some research and that perhaps we should try it. . . . If a local consultant sends patients out of hospital on a particular drug, then we tend to use it for others.'

But perhaps Dr Cracknell's most cogent comments on the prescribing habits of doctors are: 'We're a slow profession to learn. What profession isn't?' and 'We've had to learn as we go along.'

For many years now microbiologists and similar experts have

been warning against the profligate use of antibiotics for two very good reasons. The first of these is that the more that strains of antibiotic-sensitive bacteria are exposed to these agents, particularly when they are given in inadequate amounts, the more likely it is that a few antibiotic-resistant mutants within their ranks will prosper and survive and reproduce (lacking competition), so giving rise to a widespread breed of disease-producing organisms which are immune, say, to penicillin. This is already a major problem when it comes to dealing with, for example, bacterial infections of operation wounds, and it is not made easier by the fact that one species of dangerous germ can transfer its antibiotic immunity, by contact, to another. The Jeremiahs of the microbiological world have even suggested that before too long all antibiotics will become worthless unless their use is strictly and sensibly controlled, so that we'll find ourselves back in the dark ages of untreatable infections.

Second, a number of people can be rendered allergic to an antibiotic after a first dose, so that they may suffer a reaction, varying from itchiness to death, when they get a second dose. It's therefore not a very good idea to put a client at even a slight risk of being untreatable should he at some time develop pneumonia, just in order to 'cover yourself' if he comes in with a sore throat.

Dr Cracknell says that doctors took to proffering the so-called 'minor tranquillizers' (like Valium and Librium) in a big way because they were thought to be a safe substitute for the previously popular barbiturates (once a favourite means of suicide), but claims that they are now more cautiously prescribed following a realization that 'People find it difficult to get off them.'

In fact the dangers of minor tranquillizers have been recognized for some time. As far back as 1980 a British study showed that long-term users can become disturbed and confused, perhaps developing symptoms characteristic of dementia. In the same year the Department of Health issued the first of two warnings to doctors (a second being deemed necessary in 1988) drawing attention to the addictive nature of the agents, and urging that they should be prescribed for shorter periods and fewer conditions, and the US Food and Drug Administration ordered that the drugs must carry warning labels stating that they should not be used for 'anxiety or tension associated with the stress of everyday life'.

These drugs are truly addictive, meaning that habitual users not only become psychologically dependent on their 'prop', but that the biochemistry of their brains has altered to accommodate the presence of the invading ingredient, so that when it suddenly isn't there the molecular machinery doesn't function as it should, and needs time to readjust, during which period severe withdrawal symptoms may occur.

Prescriptions for tranquillizers in the UK *have* fallen, from 30.9 million in 1979 to 23.2 million in 1989, but that is still an awful lot of tranquillizers, and an estimated 1 million UK citizens are still regular (that is to say, addicted) users and are getting their supplies on the continuing say-so of their doctors, who, presumably, have either not cottoned on to or have chosen to ignore current understandings of these convenient tools.

Derek Cracknell's argument that doctors have not gone too far wrong in accepting the therapeutic advice of the pharmaceutical industry, because 'otherwise we'd have a lot more people suing us', may be in for a battering. In January 1990 more than 2,000 former British tranquillizer 'addicts' began legal proceedings against two major manufacturers of the drugs – Roche and Wyeth – on the grounds that the companies had marketed the products without reliable evidence of their safety in long-term use, and that they had failed to give adequate warnings to doctors of the risks involved. There was also talk of suing health authorities and individual prescribers.

The litigation, which is being coordinated by no fewer than 485 firms of solicitors, will be vigorously contested and will probably drag on for years. It could be disastrous if the claims succeed because countless further thousands of injured tranquillizer users might be encouraged to seek compensation, and, with a precedent set, might get it.

Good prescribing involves a good deal more than the immediate satisfaction of the immediate demands of the client on the opposite side of the surgery desk, but how many doctors recognize this truth? How many doctors had the first inkling of the possibility that in their profligate use of Valium and Librium they were creating a situation which might, just possibly, put them and their drug fountains out of business?

That's an exaggeration, of course, but doctors, who are the final arbiters of which drugs are used and how, have a massive responsibility. They are singularly ill-equipped for this responsibility, and this criticism by no means only applies to family doctors.

Some years ago I wrote a long article for *New Scientist* on the manner in which we handle modern drugs, and interviewed many people concerned with the problem. Sir Ronald Bodley-Scott, then chairman of the Medicines Commission, said to me, 'Doctors of my generation, particularly those in general practice (because hospital doctors do pick up a certain amount of information) have no idea how to use, I suppose, 90 per cent of modern drugs.' He did go on to modify that heartfelt statement by adding, 'I shouldn't say "they have no idea", because they may very well have acquired some knowledge about drugs, but at medical school they were never taught anything much in the way of clinical pharmacology or practical therapeutics.'

The late Professor James Crooks, then head of the Department of Pharmacology and Therapeutics at the University of Dundee, agreed that most doctors are not capable of handling modern drugs wisely and well, explaining this on the grounds that up until forty years or so ago physicians had hardly any effective remedies at their command, and so they concentrated upon perfecting the skills of diagnosis and prognosis.

The therapeutic revolution changed the physician's role entirely, but neither the medical curriculum nor the attitudes of practising clinicians kept pace with this change. Diagnosis is still the noblest medical skill, and treatment is still almost a secondary consideration. 'Modern drugs are such potent agents,' said Professor Crooks, 'that in order to use them rationally and effectively you really require special training.' He pointed out that only a small proportion of British medical schools had departments devoted to the study of drug treatment, 'and that even when they *are* established they usually exist only as a small appendage of the department of medicine'. The same is true in the USA. 'One trouble is that the various specialists think they know it all already,' said the professor. Thus doctors are launched into the world lacking what should have been an important part of their education, and 'so into this vacuum comes the pharmaceutical industry'.

A past president of the Royal Pharmaceutical Society, who was a dispensing chemist, bluntly described the prescribing habits of doctors as 'diabolical', and the man in the High Street pharmacy is in a good position to know what is going on. 'It's obvious,' he said, 'that you don't control the use of medicines by making them "prescription only" unless you control the people who are issuing the scrips.'

He told of a recent experience with an old man, not a regular patron of his pharmacy, who had been on three times the proper dosage of digoxin (a valuable but, in only moderate excess, potentially lethal heart drug). When the doctor responsible was contacted he said, 'Oh, God! I remember the patient. He was only supposed to be on three tablets a day for the first *week*. Change it to one a day, will you?'

Patients receiving drugs of that kind (or any drugs, for that matter) should be regularly checked so that treatment is modified to suit their changing needs, and so that a constant watch is kept for unpleasant and possibly dangerous side-effects, and the pharmacist's tale provides an example of one of the most common and least excusable causes of drug damage and misuse. This is the habit many GPs have of leaving it to their receptionists to make out repeat prescriptions for patients on long-term treatment. The doctor signs a batch of the completed forms, and the patients collect them at their leisure without bothering the boss and cluttering up an already overfilled surgery. 'We get people coming in month after month for repeat supplies of powerful drugs when they haven't been seen by the doctor for maybe five years,' said the High Street chemist.

Old people are particularly liable to suffer from lackadaisical prescribing. Ageing is likely to produce a variety of symptoms and disabilities, and doctors wedded to the 'pill for every ill' philosophy tend to employ first this remedy, then that, for the different complaints of their more ancient customers, often without realizing how the burden of medicaments is adding up. Apart from the danger of unfortunate cross-reactions or addictive effects produced by the cocktails of drugs consumed, the hapless oldies are often incapable of managing the regimens so thoughtlessly imposed upon them.

Some attempt to solve the problem of coping with their many tablets by putting them all into one bottle and shaking out the proper number at medicine time. One patient admitted to hospital under the care of Professor Crooks had a mixture of thyroid, digoxin, diuretic, potassium and sleeping pills in her pharmaceutical ditty box, and all of them were white. One day she happened to shake out five digoxin pills and suffered acute digoxin poisoning. This type of accident is a fairly frequent happening, and was described by the professor as 'a kind of pharmaceutical Russian roulette'.

A young lady house physician in a London East End hospital shared the High Street chemist's view of the prescribing habits of family doctors, saying, 'The GPs round here are terrible. Every three months they'll prescribe large batches of the drugs their patients were on when they left hospital, and without ever seeing these old people. Sooner or later they're *in extremis* once more. Then they're readmitted, and we have to start all over again.'

Another house physician, working in a London teaching hospital, had a less discouraging tale to tell, more caution being shown towards drugs by his seniors than he had expected. For example, he had soon learned that he'd be in trouble with his bosses in the morning if he'd given instructions for some treatment over the phone from his bed in the early hours, instead of getting up and seeing the patient before deciding on the proper remedy. He had also been pleasantly surprised to find that brandy was sometimes sensibly prescribed instead of sleeping tablets.

But he *had* been worried by the manner in which some of the high-powered doctors for whom he worked would give a nasty and dangerous drug to correct some abnormality which had been discovered during the course of elaborate biochemical tests, even when the nuisance caused to the patient by the fault was trivial or non-existent. Revealingly, he described a routine followed 'when a patient is looking really ill, and you're not quite sure what to do'. The drill was to withdraw all medication for twenty-four hours and see what happened. 'Sometimes patients who've been dull and drowsy and apparently on the way to death do come round. Then you realize the horrific fact that you've been poisoning them. This has happened three or four times in the past three months.'

But this was in a *teaching* hospital, one of those most sacred of temples to Aesculapius, within which the highest skills and wisdoms of the medical trade are supposedly to be found. The young lady doctor, in her ordinary NHS institution, had a more jaundiced view of her superiors. New to the trade though she was, the task of deciding what drugs patients should receive was left almost entirely in her hands, apart, that is, from the demands made by nurses for the routine prescription of sleeping tablets in the hope of ensuring a peaceful time for the staff at night. 'The surgeons don't know what to give, so they never ask you to prescribe anything. The physicians are largely interested in diagnosis, so they leave you to get on with it.' Of the three consultant physicians under whom she had served one seemed to have no interest in the drugs his patients were receiving, one was curious to know which medicines appeared to be having an effect, but only the third discussed treatment as if it was really a significant part of the business of having a patient in hospital.

This neophyte got by because most of her patients were old people suffering from heart failure, or bronchitis, or pneumonia, and the relatively few drugs she used were administered according to a standard, almost time-hallowed pattern which she remembered from her student days. 'I'm not up-to-date. We're all prescribing drugs that were prescribed ten years ago, except for the occasional novelty the consultant might have read about. I've never prescribed a drug which has been recently issued.'

And that is the quality of guidance and 'training' in the use of modern medicines which the great majority of Britain's future family doctors enjoy during the year they must work in a hospital before being licensed to go it alone. Very few graduates destined for general practice succeed in the fierce competition for house jobs within the somewhat more informed and enlightened environment of a teaching hospital. Small wonder that they fall easy prey to the seductive advertising and promotional gimmicks of the pharmaceutical industry, which becomes virtually their sole source of information concerning the products for which well over 400 million NHS prescriptions are issued each year.

The incidence of iatrogenic disease attributable to drugs is for the most part not just the unfortunate result of justifiable attempts to deal with dangerous or truly disabling complaints – that is to say, the occasional penalty to be expected from taking a calculated risk – but stems from overprescribing, and the dosing with dangerous chemicals of people who are unlikely to benefit from the nostrums so carelessly dispensed.

Admittedly, the opinions I have quoted in support of those last two condemnatory paragraphs were gathered in 1974, so I wondered whether matters have improved since then.

Dr Joe Collier says, 'The knowledge doctors have about drugs has increased enormously, but the wisdom with which they use them is probably just as questionable now as it was fifteen or twenty years ago,' and he maintains that his discipline of clinical pharmacology has so far failed to fulfil what should be its most important role – that of educating and informing people, including politicians and GPs, about the use and abuse and benefits and dangers of the powerful products of the equally powerful medicines trade. Instead, he claims, most of his colleagues have concentrated on attracting funds for research, which is often done on behalf of drug companies. 'To some extent clinical pharmacology has become the puppet of the pharmacological industry.'

This depressing view is lent credibility by the fact that in 1989 the giant American drug company, Squibb, pledged £20 million towards the cost of sustaining the Department of Pharmacology at Oxford University for five years, with the option to renew the arrangement at the end of that period. This may have been a spectacularly successful example of an academic institution acting on Mrs Thatcher's exhortation to such places to seek sponsorship from industry and other sources of private funds, but the few critics of the happening predicted that it would result in the department becoming progressively commercialized and bent upon the secret elaboration of profitable remedies, so that, once the wealthy American sugar daddy has sucked the department dry of original thought, and taken its cheque book back home, only a lifeless skeleton will remain, devoid of the capacity to pursue knowledge for its own sake, and estranged from the concept and experience of intellectual freedom. We shall see.

Indeed, we are told that progress in the healing arts would slow to an M25-type crawl but for the munificence of the drug manufacturers who now support at least 60 per cent of all medical research in universities and teaching hospitals.

It must be understood that the pharmaceutical industry is Big

Business, and its executives are not members of one of the somewhat pompously labelled 'caring professions', nominally devoted to the alleviation of human suffering, much as they might like to be so regarded in the public eye. They are tradespeople, and tradespeople of a particularly hard-nosed kind, and they are not likely to spend money on promoting understandings and attitudes which might lead to a reduced use of their wares, which is what would certainly occur if doctors were properly informed. So the major influence of the industry on medical attitudes and practice which it exerts by virtue of its purse has done nothing to improve prescribing habits.

The impression I have gained is that clinical pharmacologists have been subverted into becoming academic auxiliaries of the drug trade instead of expert advisers to the public and the medical profession.

'Read the journals,' says Joe Collier. 'It's boring old stuff which describes how drug X is absorbed this way and pissed out that way. No political issues or health issues are discussed. Clinical pharma-cology has failed in its proper purpose, mainly because of a lack of interest.' He claims to be one of the few of his fellows who regard education as a primary role, but most of them 'see what I'm doing as a waste of time, and wrong, and unacceptable'.

It has to be admitted that Joe is a bit of a maverick and iconoclast whose ideas are viewed suspiciously by many a contemporary, but that doesn't necessarily make them any the less valid. Nobody I spoke to was willing to assert that doctors *do* have a full and competent understanding of how to use drugs, and since drugs are far and away the principal weapons in the medical armamentarium, that's a pretty worrying fact.

David Ryde described a small survey he made of 100 single-item repeat prescriptions running for patients on his list. Of the total, 39 had been initiated by partners, 25 by hospital doctors, 23 by former members of the practice, 5 by former trainees attached to the practice, 1 by a district nurse, 1 by a 'stand-in', and 6 by himself. With hindsight he believed that 29 were unjustified in the first place, while the need for others was debatable. Yet all of them had been repeated over an average period of seven and a half years.

And the customers were 'hooked' on their drugs. 'Discussion with patients to review their need was largely fruitless, the consultation sometimes threatening to turn into confrontation. The book was closed. The mind made up.'

I asked Bill Grove, in his final year as a medical student, whether he had been adequately trained in the use of drugs, and what to expect from them. 'Not at all,' he said. 'I haven't a clue.' His group was taught some basic pharmacology during the pre-clinical period. The course dealt with the history and development and classes of drugs, 'but most of those described are no longer used. It was all very theoretical.'

During his clinical years Bill was expected to learn about a few agents such as contraceptives and a group of potentially dangerous heart drugs in some detail. 'But you get no general theory, and when it says "Give by slow intravenous injection", does that mean that you sit by the bed for ten minutes, or do you set up a drip, or what? Unless you've been there and seen it done you don't really know.

'We have to know the drugs and dosages used in medical emergencies. But when it actually comes, say, to using adrenaline in hospital for cardiac arrest you ask for an ampoule. It's all there on the crash trolley, and you grab the nearest thing and pump it in.'

Midway through the clinical course they had to take a multiple choice test in clinical therapeutics, but were taught nothing. Instead they had a week off other activities in which to prepare. 'So everybody gets a textbook of clinical pharmacology and reads it without really knowing what to do at all. Some people pass and some don't, and those that don't have another go. We weren't even told what text to use. They were having problems. I believe there was nobody officially in the chair of clinical pharmacology. No doubt that'll all be sorted out.'

Bill Grove expects that his future knowledge in this field will largely be derived from the handouts of the pharmacological industry.

In view of all this I was interested to know how David Ryde had, some decades since, adopted an attitude towards prescribing which is only now becoming seen as rational, and is yet to command widespread support.

'As a young family doctor I always got told off by my principals for not prescribing. It's hard to tell how this arose, and the answer is I just don't know.' So David Ryde was not *taught* the responsible use of drugs by his elders and betters in the medical trade but had to develop a sane approach to medication on his own initiative, and under the influence of experiences which even he can't certainly identify.

My impression is that not much has changed in attitudes towards drug usage since I wrote that article in 1974, except that there is now an even longer list of powerful pharmaceuticals available which can be used for better or for worse.

Heroic Surgery

Drugs are the principal but by no means the only tools of the medical trade, and other therapeutic procedures, most notably surgery, have been equally misused.

Drastic treatments are not a new phenomenon, and heroic surgery (the epithet is applied to the surgeon rather than his victim) is sometimes imposed upon patients who ought, instead, to be nursed towards a merciful death. Less traumatic surgical interventions are often employed to deal with minor or even imaginary ailments.

Commenting on ill-advised procedures, Dr Malone-Lee says, 'We're certainly taught to adopt a very optimistic attitude towards the treatments we invent. The medical literature will often promote, say, a certain operation with great enthusiasm, and ten years later its use has waned. But we're not encouraged to ask, "Why did it wane? What was wrong in the beginning that caused us to be so enthusiastic?" We're not taught to be critical of what we do and critical of how we perform, and if we do attempt to go down that road it's seen as quite a threat.'

The celebrated British surgeon, Sir Arbuthnot Lane, who died a rich man as recently as 1943, put forward the proposition, entirely without supporting evidence, that many of the ills of the flesh arise from poisons absorbed into the bloodstream from the faecal contents of the large intestine. Employing a kind of mad logic he cut out the last four or five feet of the guts of over 1,000 trusting customers in an attempt to relieve them of the probably imagined symptoms produced by the certainly imaginary toxins they were supposed to be absorbing. His clients fared better than most of the recipients of transplanted livers, and doubtless many of the survivors were convinced that the dangerous surgery had done them good, and were happy to suffer continual diarrhoea instead of the constipation which had previously been their lot.

More recently other surgical exercises of less severity but equally dubious value have been in vogue. In the 1930s between a half to three-quarters of all British children had their tonsils ripped out, often in bloody and painful 'production line' sessions, with a queue of unfortunates waiting in the corridor outside the operating theatre, new subjects being wheeled in at ten-minute intervals. Apart from the totally unnecessary pain and suffering caused to the victims of this surgical ritual, and the not infrequent tragic death from uncontrollable bleeding, an American study (in the days before mass polio immunization) revealed that after tonsillectomy children ran a four-fold increased risk of developing a particularly dangerous form of infantile paralysis. And much more recently another study has shown that people without their tonsils are three times more likely to develop Hodgkin's disease, which is a cancer of the lymph glands.

It is said that 85 per cent of the boy babies born in the USA are circumcised. Since there is no good medical reason for performing the operation on a normal penis, and since it is certain that only a tiny proportion of the infants so mutilated have been assaulted on religious grounds, we have to wonder why it happens. Unquestioning adherence to established practice, and an undue reverence for received wisdom, are important causes of many unnecessary and possibly harmful medical interventions.

Recently some surgeons have applied their minds and skills to the problem of obesity. Wiring jaws together so that compulsive eaters are forced to subsist on slops is one imaginative ploy. A Manchester surgeon has kept an inflated balloon in a customer's stomach for months on end in an attempt to curb appetite. More drastically, abdominal operations have been carried out to short-circuit great lengths of gut with the idea of preventing much of the food eaten from being absorbed.

Such simplistic mechanical approaches to what is a complex psychological and metabolic disorder take no account of the damage likely to follow from a gross interference with the normal economy of the body. They do reveal the fact that doctors who have acquired expertise as plumbers of the flesh may become bemused by their own dexterity, and that, having become mechanics, they tend to think of the human machine as an assembly of tubes and wires and parts, forgetting that each small fragment of every component is a community of microscopic cells, and that every cell is a highly active, tightly organized, precisely architectured chemical plant, and that every such cell relates, directly or indirectly, to every other. The real wonder is that so many half-thought-out surgical procedures leave those upon whom they are practised relatively unharmed.

The advent of antibiotics and many other drugs which can deal much more cheaply and much more effectively and much less traumatically with conditions which, previously, surgeons alone could tackle, deprived them of much of their *raison d'être*, so they have had to find other outlets for their skills – some (like hip and heart valve replacements) highly beneficial, some dubious.

The desire of surgeons to retain their prominent place in the medical scene could, in part, account for the present enthusiasm for all kinds of transplants. Will the fashion for these currently most glamorous of surgical conjuring tricks also wane, so that, ten or twenty years from now, we shall be wondering why they were ever performed?

The pioneer of heart transplants was, of course, the now famous Dr Christiaan Barnard, and this ultimate folly of medical prestidigitation was memorialized in an issue of the *South African Medical Journal* which appeared within days of the event. The whole magazine was devoted to the happening, and even the ads were mostly in praise of the miracle which had taken place at Groote Schuur Hospital, with messages such as 'Well done, Chris!' from the suppliers of the ligatures used, and so on.

But I treasure my copy of that issue of the magazine because it brought to marvellous life the old joke that 'the operation was a success, but the patient died'. One of the articles, signed, *inter alia*, by Christiaan Barnard, was headed 'Successful Human Heart Transplant'. On the front page of the journal, edged in black, was an announcement regretting the death of Louis Washkansky, the victim of the great experiment, who had survived the surgery for a little under three weeks.

It wasn't really a joke of course. It was a tragedy. But the death of the patient did nothing whatever to diminish the awe accorded to Dr Barnard by the world at large.

Once Barnard had taken the initiative a heart transplant epidemic spread round the world. Two transplants took place in America within forty-eight hours, then one in India, and three in quick succession in France. In May 1968 Frederick West became Britain's first heart transplant patient, and the surgical team responsible at London's National Heart Hospital held a press conference the following morning which I witnessed. The atmosphere resembled that following the defeat of the Argentinians in the Falklands. There was a total lack of serious, objective comment. The principal actors, flanked by a supporting cast of nurses, porters and technicians, waved miniature Union Jacks in the faces of the assembled mob of press, radio and television hacks who shoved, shouted and swore in the desperate competition to get 'quotes' and pictures. Frederick West died forty-six days later.

At the end of July a Mr Gordon Ford became the world's twenty-fourth and Britain's second heart transplant victim. When he died, fifty-seven hours later, only six of the remaining twenty-three were still alive, most of them having perished within days or hours.

During this heady period surgeons in Houston, Texas, put a sheep's heart into a forty-seven-year-old man who died on the spot. The British team attempted to give two dying patients pigs' hearts, and Christiaan Barnard prepared to put a baboon's heart into a five-year-old boy, but, having opened the child's chest, decided that a valve replacement would be enough to save the child's life.

There is nothing intrinsically irrational in the idea of using spare parts from other animals to replace broken-down components in Man (although I don't suppose the 'other animals' would regard the parts as 'spare'), except for the fact that the rejection problem is magnified many times, and at that stage little was known about how to handle it in the far simpler but still difficult human-to-human situation, so that these desperate ploys demonstrated a feverish anxiety among the players in the transplant extravaganza to notch up new triumphs, and attain star billing, and fast. Suitable human donors were then, and still are, rather thin on the ground, but the surgeons couldn't wait.

Artificial hearts have enjoyed a brief vogue within the recent past because contraptions made of metal and plastic are clearly not subject to destruction by the body's defence mechanisms, and so might be expected to prove the answer to the transplanters' greatest apparent problem.

Several attempts at replacing the entire heart with a permanent implant, necessarily connected by tubes emerging from the chest to a massive power unit, have only succeeded in keeping the unfortunate recipients alive for periods ranging from days to months, but shackled to their immovable machines, and in an increasingly wretched state. They have commonly suffered and finally succumbed to a series of strokes caused by blood clots forming in the implant before breaking loose and lodging in the brain.

A small band of enthusiasts continue to experiment, and believe that new materials and techniques will eventually lead to the development of satisfactory instruments, including circulation boosters, or auxiliary pumps, designed to provide temporary assistance to the failing natural organ, giving it a chance to recover, or perhaps just keeping the patient going until a suitable donor heart should become available.

But the use of such appliances must still, I maintain, be regarded as an unjustifiable use of the desperately ill as experimental animals, and an example of an all-too-common failure to recognize that a duty to serve the best interests of the individual patient should always override an intrinsically worthy ambition to advance medical technology, let alone the far less worthy purpose of advancing the experimenter's own reputation.

Meanwhile the enthusiasm for heart and heart-and-lung and liver transplants continues, because (in contrast to the artificial heart adventure) a proportion of the recipients of natural spare parts survive, and in better health, for at least a time.

It's dramatic. It's up there on the front line of the curative assault upon disease, offering an instant solution to a serious problem, but does it pay dividends?

A fact not given much publicity is that patients near to death because of a failing heart (particularly a dilated cardiomyopathy, which is the principal indication for a heart transplant) do at least as well if left to the physicians as if they had been serviced by the surgeons. On either routine about two-thirds last a year and a little more than one-third last for five.

This being so, it could be argued that some kinds of transplant should be abandoned on the simple grounds that they have not added anything to the hope for life, and that they cost an awful lot of money, and that the need to 'harvest' organs from the 'near-dead' or so-called 'brain-dead' has raised a set of ethical and legal problems we could well do without.

Some transplants (like corneas and blood) are acceptable because they work well and can solve a problem. Others aren't because they clearly can't.

That's why I call heart (let alone liver) transplants bad medicine, because they can never make more than an insignificant impact upon the toll of premature death and suffering exacted by heart disease, and their cost in terms of the money and effort involved is grotesquely disproportionate to any dubious good they could ever do to a tiny proportion of cardiac invalids.

Kidney transplants are a less evidently futile exercise for two main reasons. In the first place, far fewer people face death each year from kidney failure than the number who perish from heart disease. In Britain it is something like 2,000 compared to 170,000, and of the 2,000 only some 60 per cent are deemed suitable for treatment. So, if the technique, and particularly the post-operative management routine, could be so improved that every transplant restored to the recipient a normal life expectancy (and a life of good quality to boot), a cure could be provided for everyone who might benefit from the exercise. Four transplants a day, with no weekend work, would settle the matter. Second, people without working kidneys can be kept alive and reasonably active by the use of kidney machines, to which they have to be connected twice or thrice a week for several hours.

These machines were once regarded as the answer to the kidney failure problem, but their use does impose severe limitations on the freedom of the patients, who also have to stick to a somewhat tedious diet, and many of them never feel really fit. However, the availability of the machine is a great help to the transplant surgeons. Ill patients can be restored to reasonable health before an operation, so that their chances of surviving the immediate trauma are improved. They can be kept well for months or even years until a fresh, well-matched kidney becomes available, so that the need to take risks with less well-matched organs is avoided. Most importantly, if a transplanted kidney fails, the patient does not die but is put back on a machine to await a second operation. Some patients receive three or four new kidneys over a period of time.

Transplants, combined with the use of machines, do postpone the deaths of around 1,000 UK citizens annually, who then survive for varying periods, and often for several years, but about 20 per cent of transplanted kidneys don't even start functioning. 'Good' results are only obtained at certain centres of excellence where a great deal of time, skill and money have been applied to improving the management of patients, so that whereas over 80 per cent of grafts last for three months in the best hands, only 14 per cent last that long in the worst.

So transplantation is far from being the once-and-for-all salvage operation (which the propagandists tend to suggest it is), after which the lucky recipients can forget their troubles and rejoin the herd. They are permanently on anti-rejection drugs which increase their susceptibility to infections and even to cancer. They face the prospect of repeated major surgery interspersed by spells on a kidney machine. Some patients do enjoy substantial interludes of well-being, but others are anxious, below par and depressed, and find the extra life they have been given burdensome.

Bill Grove, the final year student, told me of a cousin who had died recently from a kidney disease. 'She'd been run through the medical mill. She'd had two kidney transplants, and had been experimented on, and died a very sad and miserable person, and the medical profession had had great fun with her.

'A classic question at interviews for medical school is "What do you think of heart transplants?" The "right" answer is, "Ah well, they're like kidneys were fifteen years ago. In fifteen years' time hearts will be as good as kidneys". But I say to that, kidney transplants aren't good either, because although it's technically a very easy operation now, and you give drugs so that by and large the organs aren't rejected, and there's an 80 per cent five-year survival rate with live donors, and so on, a lot of these people have really miserable lives, and that's just not on.

'It's so self-centred for the medical profession to sit back and say, "We can do kidney transplants, and they're great" when people are suffering complete misery, and would have been much better off if they'd died.'

Unfortunately, while all this costly, hi-tech rescue work is being pursued with immense enthusiasm, energy, dedication and skill by some of our ablest and most influential doctors, less glamorous but potentially much more effective measures available for reducing the toll exacted by heart, liver and kidney disease are given a low priority.

In 1989, for example, the National Kidney Research Fund claimed, on good evidence, that one in ten cases of kidney failure could be prevented if family doctors made a routine check for high blood pressure in their patients and took steps to reduce it. And in a separate report from University College Hospital, London, it was stated that one in five cases of kidney failure in teenagers and adults could be prevented if GPs made a practice of sending a urine sample for analysis whenever they suspected the common condition of urinary tract infection in their young patients, and then treated confirmed cases with a short course of an antibiotic. So here are two cheap and easy measures which, conscientiously applied, could, together, cut the 'need' for kidney transplants by a wondrous 30 per cent.

Such simple procedures would, in no measurable manner, divert doctors from the task of helping the already gravely ill. They would, indeed, give them more time to devote to such unfortunates, because there would be fewer of them.

Never Say 'Die'

Doctors not only seem to prefer to invent and practise techniques for salvaging the dangerously ill, rather than concentrating on the more sensible task of preventing their clients from becoming dangerously ill in the first place, they are also reluctant to 'let go' when a patient is beyond any reasonable hope of responding to whatever curative help they can offer.

General Franco of Spain, President Tito of Yugoslavia and the Emperor Hirohito of Japan, have been well-publicized examples of the terminally ill who have been subjected to horrific procedures in a cruel attempt to keep them 'alive' well after the Grim Reaper had announced that their time was up. It may be that political considerations inspired some of these abuses of the medical craft, but you don't have to be a head of state to attract this kind of attention.

Some years ago a friend of mine in her forties developed cancer of the ovary. She was a cheerful, vigorous, hard-working jewel of a woman who raised the spirits of everybody she dealt with. Her breakdown was sudden. One day she was about her usual business, and the next she suffered acute abdominal pain and was taken to hospital. The pain soon disappeared and never returned, but over the course of the next eight weeks or so she became progressively weaker and thinner and, most importantly, more and more discouraged.

Her cancer was inoperable. She was given chemotherapy. The pills made her sick and wretched far beyond any malaise that might be blamed on the disorder they were supposed to attack. She knew they were causing much of the distress and misery she felt, but, home again from hospital for a while, she faithfully and courageously swallowed the sickening tablets because of the hope held out to her that they would purge the poison in her belly, and put her back on her feet again, and let her return to the job and associates she so clearly loved.

I say 'the hope held out to her' because I don't believe she ever really felt that hope herself. She said to me, once or twice in her sad time, 'They should have just let me go and have done with it.' And she asked me more than once, 'Are they doing me good? Are they going to work?'

When she said these things I was with her as a friend, and not as her medical advisor, and since I didn't know exactly what she had been told, and since I knew I could only cause further worry and distress by contradicting whatever information she may have been given, I could not say what I believed, and I made such comforting and encouraging sounds as I was able to summon up, but felt my words were futile.

After three or four weeks at home she was moved back to hospital for the constant nursing care she had come to need. The pills she had come to fear and dislike so much were stopped a week or ten days before she died.

I don't believe she was ever told of her true state, and she was encouraged to think that the sickness engendered by the hated tablets must be endured because they could cure her disease. But I think that from the first she knew in her heart she was doomed, and I think she suspected, also, that she had to tolerate her distressing treatment more for her doctors' sakes than for her own.

Bill Grove had a similar tale to tell. 'Even now, when the quality of life is supposed to be important, I've seen women riddled with breast cancer who have no chest left – just one great fungating ulcerating mass – and you're piling in chemotherapeutic agents and telling them, "Maybe you'll get better," when they're obviously on the verge of death.

'We had a patient just like that, and I felt that what she needed was to be told, "You're going to die" so that she could come to terms with it, and tell her young family what was going on, and say goodbye to her husband and young children. But they said, "No. We'll give you another course of therapy." I argued with the consultant afterwards and he was very angry with me and said, "If you look at the statistics you'll find that one in a thousand patients in this condition will pull through with the drug, so I can't tell her she's bound to die." She was dead the following morning, and hadn't been given the opportunity to come to terms with what was happening to her.'

These are not unusual stories. Too many cancer patients have their last days or weeks or months made wretched by intensive treatment with drugs or radiation or surgery or all three when there is no reasonable prospect of a cure, and when they should have been allowed to die in dignity and peace.

Why does this happen? In part, perhaps, because the experts involved are unwilling to admit helplessness and defeat, and feel that they have to take some kind of aggressive action in the face of impending death. But there is a less emotional and, one might almost say, more cynical reason. The patients so treated (just like the recipients of artificial hearts) are, to put the matter brutally, being used as experimental animals, and are being subjected to therapy with known ill effects, not in the reasonable expectation that their lives can be saved, but because of a felt need to try this approach and that to a so far unsolved problem in the hope that, eventually, a regime will be found that does relieve the distress and prolong the lives of future victims of the same disease.

Mrs Wendy Savage, the outspoken consultant obstetrician who won unwanted national fame when she was unrightfully suspended from her job because of a disreputable internecine dispute at the London Hospital, says, 'Factors which influence the quality of people's lives, like the sort of care provided for the mentally ill and handicapped, are always low down on the list of priorities for doctors. Doctors who get to a position where they can influence things are much more interested in the exciting cutting edges like cardiac surgery or *in vitro* fertilization.

'I saw a marvellous example of this in Russia – the place where they can't even manufacture the sheath and distribute it to the population, so that women are having five or six abortions for every live birth. And there we went to see somebody doing IVF. I found it quite extraordinary. There they were, with hospitals thirty-five years out-of-date by our standards, and yet they were wanting to get on to this IVF bandwagon.

'The professor concerned said, "You've got to allow for the high-flyers."

'I said, "If the high-flyers weren't going off into these flights of fancy, maybe they could put their minds to such simple things as to how to distribute the sheath, and make it so that it doesn't break."

'That seems to be a fundamental problem and flaw in our training. People are trained in such a competitive way, with all these hurdles to leap over, and they're lost if they don't *have* hurdles once they get into their practical work.'

Rabbi Julia Neuberger, who has become an authority on health care matters and who is Chairman of the Patients Association, says, 'Doctors are taught to cure, and, unless they're actually working in terminal care, they still find it very hard to say, "We cannot do anything." The result is that they continue to treat unnecessarily. That can be very cruel. But they do it because their whole philosophy is directed towards cure rather than care.

'Therefore other people should be involved in creating the philosophy, and asking whether it should be directed just towards cure, or should also involve caring, palliative treatment, which one sees at its best at hospices, and the Royal Marsden, and the Marie Curie Foundation, and so on.

'Then there'd be a whole different ball game, and some of the treatments would change. AIDS patients should get the same kind of care as any others, with no questions asked, but they don't, because of the politics of AIDS.'

Wendy Savage mentions an additional cause of the sometimes infelicitous manner in which hospital doctors handle their customers.

'It's so difficult when you're working in hospital to maintain your understanding of the psychological aspects of disease, because it's all so episodic. And now – the way the infrastructure's been destroyed – it's so difficult to do a ward round in which you can think. The notes aren't there, and there's nobody to go round with you, and nobody knows the patient, and the ward's in a mess, and it's noisy, and the phone keeps on ringing, and the house officer's bleep keeps going. It's just like a nightmare sometimes.'

Why Do It?

I asked Dr Malone-Lee why he had chosen geriatrics as his specialty.

'I made the choice while I was in the Army. I'd intended to be a GP and then got pushed into becoming a physician. I had my membership [MRCP – the competitive and demanding higher qualification which all aspiring physicians must achieve] and had done a general medical registrar training job, which included quite a lot of neurology. I started looking at the NHS in the run-up to the time that I was due to leave the Army, and got the impression that there were a lot of medical specialties which seemed to be cluttered up with dashing young doctors, all desperately trying to make it, and none of it looked terribly challenging. I thought I'd be spending my time trying to look enthusiastic over rather trivial aspects of care which I wouldn't feel very comfortable with, so I looked around for something dirty and difficult, and geriatrics was one such field.

'I'd seen a lot of neurology with people getting enthusiastic about rare conditions, when the bulk of patients don't have such conditions. I wanted to get into something where things weren't happening or hadn't happened, and which was difficult, and would be a challenge. Geriatrics was pretty ropy then, at the beginning of the '80s.

'It's been fantastic. Better than my wildest dreams. I never realized it was going to be so attractive. And I'm confident for the future. I've got another twenty-five years or so to go, but I don't think I'm going to be bored in that time, or that there aren't going to be many more challenges.'

I asked whether geriatrics was beginning to emerge from the shadow of being regarded as a Cinderella specialty.

'I'm quite happy for it to be regarded as a Cinderella specialty by the sort of people who make that kind of remark. I don't actually *want* to be respected by those people.'

I asked Ellis Downes, the newly qualified doctor, why he had decided on a career in obstetrics and gynaecology.

'Because it's an all-round specialty. There's some surgery (I love surgery, but I could never do hernias until I'm sixty). There's also some medicine and some endocrinology and there are plenty of opportunities for research (I'm particularly interested in infertility). But the ultimate thing is that most patients are fairly fit and young, and you can talk to and relate to them very well. There's counselling and contraception. It just seems to have an awful lot in it.

'And it's a fairly happy specialty most of the time. You get your tragedies, with babies who die, and so on, but on the whole it's a happy, jolly specialty. Very few patients die, which is nice, and unlike the situation in, say, general medicine or geriatrics.

'We all have different niches. Every doctor finds something which presents a personal challenge. For me it's the challenge of being able to help a couple who can't have children to have children. I can't think of anything greater for a doctor to do.'

It is just as well that the profession attracts men and women of widely differing aptitudes and attitudes, for there are so many widely differing tasks to be done. There is no lack of challenging problems. The need is somehow to persuade our cleverest doctors to devote their energies to the practice of the best kind of medicine. And with finite resources but an infinite demand this must mean medicine of a kind which pays good dividends in terms of the prevention and relief of suffering.

Some of the means being developed in an attempt to achieve this end are discussed in Chapter 5. Meanwhile, let the last word on the theme of doctors and disease go to Bill Grove, the final year student.

'Doctors are not there to satisfy their ego.'

4 Doctors and Patients

David Ryde, the parsimonious prescriber, has lambently described the three stages he believes doctors go through in their attitude towards their patients while they (the doctors) are on their way to a state of professional maturity.

These he has labelled sympathy, empathy and apathy.

To begin with the young doctor feels an emotional involvement with his patients as he enjoys the novelty of being accepted as a recipient of their most intimate feelings and problems. With a little more experience he begins to get a better understanding of the nature of those problems, and views them with comprehension but 'detached concern'. However, and all too soon, the doctor's response to his customers' complaints becomes a matter of 'polite indifference', because 'We've all seen it so often before that we become insensitive to the patient's feelings and message.'

Dr Ryde's assessment of the progress of his fellow practitioners' attitudes toward their patients would, I am sure, elicit growls of agreement from some and shouts of denial from others, but I have gained the impression that a lot of doctors do regard their patrons as awkward customers who tend to expect too much of their medical advisors.

Dr Cracknell, who has spent some forty years in general practice, harks back to the days when the doctor's word was law. 'You had the expertise. People would listen to you. They wouldn't question you. They'd say, "You're the doctor, I'm the patient. I have the pain. You tell me what it is. Give me something and I'll go away."

'Now they're more likely to come and say, "I've looked up my textbook, and it tells me it might be this, that or the other. What do you think?" That's the different approach we're getting from patients. So we say, "Right – I've examined you, and I'm going to do the following tests, and when I get the results you come back and we'll discuss the appropriate line of treatment." Then they're going to say, "Why do you think this is better than that?" or "Joe Bloggs down the road had so-and-so from his doctor for the same sort of thing. Why aren't you giving me that?" That's happening much more now than ever before.' (It is significant that the BMA *Family Health Encyclopaedia*, published last year, which describes the nature, symptoms and treatment of practically every known disease, leapt into the bestseller charts despite its daunting cover price of £25.)

Not only does Dr Cracknell find his patients less subservient and more likely to question the medical fiat than heretofore – they also have higher expectations.

'Papers and magazines encourage readers to go along to doctors and demand this, that and the other, but there *is* no automatic right to things.' The media often seem to get the blame when people don't behave in the way that other people think they should, but Dr Cracknell concedes that the medical profession is also itself partly responsible for the increased pressures being put upon it. 'We have acquiesced to the popular demand that the doctor will cure.'

Revealingly, he followed that remark by a specific and apparently trivial complaint. 'Because children get their prescriptions free, every cough medicine is provided by the doctor instead of the patient going straight to the chemist. If you are hard up or have a big family it's much better to go to the doctor. It may only save you 50p or £1, but while you're passing your doctor's door you might as well call in and get it.'

Now, it is generally agreed amongst the pharmacological cognoscenti that 'cough medicines' in general are pretty useless, and sometimes positively harmful when a powerful agent, truly capable of suppressing the cough reflex, is employed to diminish the hawking out of phlegm. So Dr Cracknell is railing against the fact that 'the system' (the NHS, which encourages his clients to believe that they have a right to a remedy for every ill) is forcing him to prescribe medicines he doesn't believe in to patients who don't need them. 'Kevin has a cough. Do something about it. I pay my taxes, don't I?'

Perhaps the label of David Ryde's third stage of 'apathy' should be changed to describe a rather more active emotion, such as 'irritation' or 'resentment'. I suppose it depends on the temperament of the individual doctor. But one thing seems clear. Many if not most doctors feel that their customers do not appreciate what doctors are for, and there is a common notion that the public must be 'educated' in the use of the services available, and stop cluttering up surgery waiting rooms and out-patient departments in a vain search for a solution to problems which they ought to deal with themselves, or which they shouldn't have allowed to develop, or which ought to be the responsibility of other agencies.

Dr John Marks, speaking as a GP rather than as Chairman of the BMA, says that 'A large number of the patients we see present with emotional problems which we can't solve for them. They really need a new husband or a different house. We can't provide those.'

So it would appear that a considerable part of the discontent which doctors (specially general practitioners) feel in regard to their dealings with patients lies in the fact that they are not equipped or empowered to deal with many of their customers' true needs, which is frustrating for both the providers and consumers of care. I have not heard lawyers or accountants or generals complain in this fashion (except that generals would always like more guns and tanks), but I suspect that many a clergyman and schoolteacher must often feel the same way.

Hospital doctors may not suffer the same kind of frustrations as GPs (except to the extent that they may feel themselves hampered by lack of money or supporting staff or beds), because, in general, they only see people whom family doctors have already identified as being in need of the help which a particular specialty can offer. Therefore they are less likely to be confronted by patients who they feel shouldn't have bothered them in the first place, or who present with problems they can't do very much about. But this means that they are the more likely to regard their customers as the vehicles of a disease rather than as people with emotions and a host of practical, everyday demands to deal with, and for whom illness is only an extra and often frightening difficulty added to an already difficult life.

'I've dealt with your complaint in the approved fashion, and that's an end to the matter. A pat on the back for all concerned. Goodbye.' Or, even less happily, 'This is a very interesting but obstinate condition, and we must have you in and try this, that and the next thing, and we can't let you remove your disease from our juris-diction until we've finished with it.' And never mind what all the investigations and therapies and instructions may mean in terms of a disrupted life and mental turmoil for the 'carriers' of a fault of the flesh or of the mind, and for their families.

George Teeling Smith says, 'It is novel for the majority of doctors to worry about how the patient feels and can function after you've treated him, rather than just judging whether "the operation's a success" the day after you've done it.'

Derek Cracknell says, 'We need to recognize that people in the community have to cope with life not only in the family, but also in the workplace and so on. I can think of many instances such as, say, an orthopaedic surgeon telling a man whose job involves climbing up and down ladders that he's now fit for work. The surgeon never found out what the man's job was, except that he worked in a factory, and he's ended up with a straight leg, and there's no way you can climb ladders with a straight leg.'

'We treat people's symptoms,' comments Ellis Downes. 'For example, I treat a miscarriage to stop the haemorrhage, but do I think about the death of the baby and what it means to the woman and her partner? Or a woman comes in with a broken leg. What are the implications of six weeks off work? We forget that. We're not interested. We just make certain the lady's physical fault is dealt with properly, and review the outcome in six weeks' time to make sure it's healed properly. As doctors we're not sufficiently interested in the patient's welfare, and it's a gross indictment of medical schools that we haven't educated doctors to take that on board. A lot of doctors say, "That's not my job. My job is to set the knee and get them out of hospital." I disagree. We *should* care. Doctors aren't adopting the holistic approach enough – treating minds as well as bodies.'

Bill Grove described an exchange he'd recently witnessed between a surgeon and a woman with a kidney cancer. She had asked whether the suggested removal of the organ was really going to improve her lot, and the surgeon had replied, 'I have to imagine you're my mother, and think what I'd say to her.' 'Very few people think like that,' said Grove, 'but those who do are the ones I most admire.'

The apparently encouraging thing is that the views expressed by these four, and most feelingly by the two youngest of them, were echoed by most of my other respondents. These views are becoming increasingly widely held, so it may be that more of the next generation of patients will find a more supportive and understanding response when they're unlucky enough to have to seek medical aid.

On the other hand, of course, it might be that the two young people quoted were still locked into David Ryde's stage one of sympathy, and will later discover that apathy or irritation or frustration take over, or that it is simply very much easier to concentrate upon the disease and to neglect the problems posed by the person. And perhaps their older colleagues were only paying lip service to a concept of the nature of good medical care which has been popularized by outside critics of the medical scene like economists and sociologists and journalists and politicians and consumer groups, all of whom can see what appears to be wrong, but who have never had to cope with the front-line strains and stresses of medical practice.

Perhaps it is unrealistic to expect any but a few exceptional men and women (and most doctors are fairly ordinary people) to manage to be all things to all men over the course of a professional lifetime.

Professor Bosanquet suggests, for example, that NHS consultants tend to be burned out before they even start. 'They are tired after the ten to fifteen years' very, very hard work involved in becoming a consultant, and feel themselves overwhelmed by the large machine of a modern hospital. In a sense consultants' careers are now affected by the sheer size and capital stock of the machine and the hospital system. There's less sense of the individual being able to carve out something distinctive and to be something distinctive.

'There is the feeling that hospital doctors are anchored in an inland sea which is rapidly drying out. There isn't the money – either capital or revenue – to support the kind of hardware and the kind of service level they've been given in the past. They don't have a clear philosophy of the patient as a whole person, and what their contribution is doing to the welfare of the patient as a whole person. They tend to be over-specialized.'

Small wonder, then, if some of our more able and ambitious hospital doctors endeavour to 'use' their patients as a means for demonstrating their own professional skills and worthiness, instead of considering, first, whether a new or adventurous and impressive procedure is truly likely to be in those patients' best interests.

It's a complex and complicated business, this relationship between the doctor and his patient, which can be influenced by many emotional and irrational factors, and is not always based on a cool, logical and informed analysis of the circumstances surrounding each encounter.

I asked Ra Gillon, who had said that the prime job of doctors is to help people who are ill, whether he could define the nature of the contract between the doctor and his client, and whether he liked the term 'patient'.

He said, 'Yes. It's a very important term. On the other hand, what I like about the notion of the term "client" is that it implies that patients are independent, autonomous agents, and must always be regarded as that, except in the few cases where they actually aren't, and we have to have ways of dealing with that.

'For the most part people *are* independent, autonomous agents, and the only reason a doctor has been allowed to get his mitts on them is because they've asked for it. Again, there are a few exceptions, either because they're so severely ill that they're no longer adequately autonomous agents able to look after their own affairs, or because they're so severely ill that they're endangering other people.

'Otherwise the relationship has always been based on the desire of the patient to come and get medical help, and as soon as that breaks down – piss off!'

Taking that situation as the norm, Dr Gillon went on to say that doctors should be prepared to justify any *imposition* of 'help' when help has not been asked for and is not wanted.

'It's only very recently that there has been any question of people being treated against their will. There just weren't enough medical resources around, so that even people who wanted medical treatment were jolly lucky if they could get it. That's why there's been no emphasis on people's autonomy, because it's been implicit.'

He had in mind, I suppose, the imposition of treatment on patients 'for their own good' (as, for example, the sterilization of mentally subnormal girls judged incapable of coping with motherhood), because, of course, unfortunates like 'dangerous' lunatics or smallpox victims have long been subjected to compulsory 'treatment' in the interests of the community at large. But, that apart, I suggested that the very jargon surrounding the doctor–patient relationship hardly supports the idea of a longstanding implicit acknowledgment of the customer's autonomy. Patients are 'under doctors' orders' and are 'forbidden' this or 'allowed' that and are 'detained in' or 'released from' hospital.

'I don't know when this started,' said Gillon, 'but I suspect that the more medicine has become institutionalized and a part of the State system, the more it has become a problem. But to talk about "doctors' orders" is a mistake. A lot of people when asking advice from an expert are prepared to say, 'Tell me what to do, and I'll do it." That's a perfectly respectable thing to do so long as you do it deliberately and willingly. That's entirely "autonomy-respecting". If I take a car to the garage and say, "Service it – do what's necessary", that's fine. That's an implicit agreement which can, if necessary, become explicit. But if doing what's necessary looks like becoming too expensive in one sense or another, then I say, "Ring me – let me decide." That analogy's quite appropriate to medicine.

'You've got all sorts of implicit agreements. You don't have to go through the whole formal rigmarole of asking permission to choose whether to use erythromycin rather than penicillin, for example. But if I wanted to treat somebody with a substantially more dangerous drug, because I thought it was more appropriate in that case, I'd say, "I don't think penicillin is going to help here. The only thing which has a chance of helping is something quite dangerous." So you need to work out the pros and cons of that. "You, the patient, can choose, or you can leave it to me. But that's for you to decide."

'Also, when you're spending other people's money, you have to take into account whether that money would be better spent on that patient or other potential patients.'

My own impression is that the central importance of doctors acknowledging their patients' autonomy, so that they, the doctors, modify their actions and attitudes in the light of such acknowledgment, has only recently become a fashionable concept, largely generated from outside the profession. Insiders, like Ra Gillon and James Malone-Lee and Wendy Savage and, now, many others, who are demanding that their colleagues keep a critical eye on what they are doing and why, are a new and encouraging phenomenon. Hitherto doctors (just like lawyers) have been enormously self-satisfied, and fellow members of the guild who criticize this complacency have been, and too often, still are, regarded as mavericks and a threat.

So I don't agree with Dr Gillon when he suggests that the concept of the autonomy of the patient has not, until recently, been actively argued and examined because it was accepted and implied. It hasn't been discussed because it didn't exist. Certainly when I was a medical student at St Thomas' Hospital in London, some fifty years ago, the authority of the doctor over the patient (be it the consultant in the ward or out-patient clinic, or the tyro dealing with customers in the casualty department) could not, conceivably, be questioned. Once within the portals the patients had surrendered themselves to the medical will, and any expression of questioning or discontent was commonly and promptly suppressed by domineering sisters who knew just how to keep rebellious-minded patients in their proper place, so that the doctors were commonly shielded from even an awareness that their ministrations might be being less than happily received.

At St Thomas', at that time, the patients were little more than medical cannon-fodder. The atmosphere of the place encouraged us to regard the people we were there to serve as ignorant peasants who had to be handled with the kind of paternalistic discipline to be expected in a home for wayward boys. Not much evidence of an implicit acknowledgment of the patient's autonomy there, and I suppose the attitudes bred stuck with many who went through that kind of apprenticeship for the rest of their careers.

Have things changed much since then?

Margaret Martin is Secretary of the Cambridge Community Health Council. (The role of CHCs is discussed below, see page 75.) She has firm views on the relationship existing between doctors and their clients today.

'When you don't need doctors they're part of the professional network which will include bank managers and all the other professionals we deal with. But when you do need them they suddenly change into almost God-like people, and you don't relate to them in the way that you relate to other professionals.

'I wouldn't say to my bank manager, "Look after my money. Don't tell me what's in my account. I know it's safe in your hands." It's my money and I want to be in charge of it. But with doctors we totally change our approach. Once you require a doctor's services you become very needy and vulnerable and go along cap in hand. When I go to the doctor I have to fight against my own sense of vulnerability. This is the difficulty, and doctors don't always help because they're used to being put on a pedestal and having all that power over life and death and our basic needs.

'It can intoxicate, and make them feel powerful, and encourage people to treat them in that very subservient way instead of as partners.'

Margaret Martin later stressed the importance of that last remark. 'Every single one of the things that go wrong, and which bring people here, could be put down to the doctor's or patient's lack of understanding of the fact that their relationship is one of partnership.'

A commonly heard complaint from patients is that their doctors don't tell them anything. They don't communicate. Numerous studies have shown that many people leaving surgeries or outpatient departments retain only a partial or confused memory of the advice and instructions which their medical counsellors believe they have provided.

That could be because so many of us are a bit thick.

Or it could be because doctors are pretty bad at issuing advice in terms which the medically illiterate (that's most of us) can understand.

Or it could be because doctors don't even attempt to explain what's really going on because they have been taught to deal with disease rather than people, and so regard their assessment of a customer's condition as something beyond that customer's comprehension, and within their province alone, and don't see the effort of explaining what's going on as relevant to their task.

Julia Neuberger agreed that this is part of the problem. 'If the whole of your education is disease-oriented, which is what hospital medicine does for you, then you don't think about people. You think of the patient as a scientific problem. There's a problem in this body. This part has gone wrong. It's like a car. People don't talk to a car, and doctors don't talk to patients either.' But she went on to express the belief that a more fundamental reason for poor communication is that doctors are imitating a consulting room or bedside manner which they've been brought up to regard as orthodox and proper. 'They simply copy what everybody else has always done.'

The encouraging fact is that the problem is now widely acknowledged, not only by the patients who are on the receiving end, but by doctors themselves, and efforts are being made to teach communication skills, which can be done effectively, as by videotaping real or acted consultations and playing the results back to the doctors concerned. 'Sometimes when you use this technique and show people what they're actually doing they're appalled, because they don't even know they're doing it,' says Rabbi Neuberger. 'It ought to be much more widely used.'

James Malone-Lee has demonstrated that involving his patients in as full an understanding as possible of what he is trying to do for them not only makes them happier and more cooperative partners in the therapeutic effort, but may actually lead to a marked improvement in the handling of their complaints.

He runs an incontinence clinic. Having a leaky bladder doesn't kill you, but it is a damned distressing and depressing business which medicines can alleviate. 'I have three potentially helpful drugs at my disposal, and the makers tell me the doses I should prescribe. We've found that if we ask the patients to manage their own medication, and to alter the dosage according to the way they're responding and how they think they ought to take their pills, then we can achieve effective responses using dose schedules which the manufacturers never thought were appropriate. . . . I wouldn't have found that out without giving patients the freedom to work it out for themselves. And giving them control of the therapy is not very threatening at all.'

The lesson here, it seems to me, is that patients often understand more about the way a prescribed course of action is affecting their well-being than their doctors do, and that *talking with* rather than simply *instructing* their customers (quite apart from the small matter of respecting their clients' dignity and 'autonomy') can give doctors a better chance of doing a good job.

Margaret Martin is absolutely on the ball when she claims that a lack of a sense of partnership is the principal cause of discontent between the profession and the people it serves. But a sense of partnership must involve some kind of emotional attachment, and I asked Ra Gillon whether he could identify the ideal emotional relationship that should exist between a doctor and his patient. He referred me to 'a very nice book' called *Moderated Love* by Alistair Campbell. The author's theme is that ordinary love, such as for a husband, lover, wife or child, isn't the appropriate emotion in any professional relationship. On the other hand, neither is the ordinary detachment you have to any other member of society. Campbell goes for a position in between, which he calls 'moderated love'. So the emotion of love informs the relationship, but so does the detachment, and the combination allows for a critical and effectual assessment and management of the affiliation, as opposed to the unqualified commitment demanded by total love.

I suspect that many doctors would experience embarrassment or even anger at the suggestion that love, even if it *is* 'moderated love', is an element in every fruitful doctor–patient relationship (a reaction that might spring, in part, from an allergy to the word because of the fact that any overt emotional entanglement with a patient has always been near the top of the list of cardinal medical sins). But I also suspect that where love is absent the partnership is likely to be sterile, and the outcome less than satisfactory, and that the best doctors are in the first division of their craft precisely because they do allow love to moderate their attitudes and actions, and not just because they are clever medical technicians.

It is a regrettable but well-researched and documented fact that some of us stand a far better chance of enjoying good health, and of receiving the best available medical care when health breaks down, than others.

Inequalities of health care are not nearly so marked here in the UK as they are, for example, in the ultra-free market system of medicine operating in the USA, where, because of the limited cover provided by expensive medical insurance, prosperous families can be reduced to penury by the costs of a serious illness in one of its members, and where the old and the poor get, at best, a grudgingly provided second-class service, and where Thomas Burke, a former chief of staff of the Department of Health and Human Services in the Reagan administration, recently felt moved to say that 'The doctors in this country are ripping us off blind with excessive costs and unnecessary treatments.' But why should gross inequalities prevail here in the UK – this happy, welfare state?

Why, for example, during 1986–8, should perinatal deaths (the number of babies dying at birth or within the first week of life) have occurred at the rate of 13.5 per 1,000 live births at Bradford in Yorkshire, but only at 5.1 per 1,000 at Huntingdon in Cambridgeshire? In England heart disease is responsible for more than a quarter of all deaths (which fact, in itself, is bad enough, considering that much of it is preventable), but why should the death rate from cardiac problems be between 30–50 per cent higher than the national average in parts of the industrial north, and well below that average in places like Kingston upon Thames and Esher in prosperous Surrey?

Clearly life-style, the quality of housing and nutrition, stresses of debt and unemployment, perhaps racial harassment, and similar social factors contribute to the differences. 'The most important remedy for poor health in inner city areas is to reduce inequalities of income and life opportunities in general,' says Professor Bosanquet. 'It's doubtful how far the health services can influence the problem, and we may be deluding ourselves in thinking they can.'

Julia Neuberger agrees. 'This is a British problem, and you can argue over the extent to which it's a problem for the medical profession *per se*, or a much wider social policy issue.' She singles out poor housing, poor nutrition and a lack of control over conditions in the workplace (the tardy response to the toll exacted by pneumoconiosis and industrial accidents, for example) as instances of circumstances favouring disease which governments can influence and doctors can't do much about.

She doesn't, however, let doctors off the hook entirely. 'Poor diet is something that you can, to some extent, blame on the medical profession, because we have such a poor record of health education and health promotion.' But even in this matter she wouldn't 'necessarily blame the GP' because health promotion is so poorly funded and needs 'a much more massive campaign than the Government is prepared to pay for'. And she concludes that 'there are massive inequalities in health care which I wouldn't particularly blame on the medical profession.'

But given the fact that governments rather than doctors are best placed to iron out the grosser inequalities in the prospects for a healthy life, do doctors do all that they can to improve matters?

Rabbi Neuberger comments on the different treatment offered by GPs and hospital doctors to middle-class patients as compared to the manner in which they deal with clients from the working class. 'It is a marked tendency in out-patient departments for middle-class patients to be shoved to the head of the queue, and to be seen more quickly, and for consultants to spend slightly more time with middle-class rather than working-class patients. I don't think that doctors are any different from any other profession in that respect. It's the same with teachers and lawyers. It's a universal problem with professionals, who are middle-class themselves, and have difficulty in relating to people who aren't. That says more about British society than it does about the medical profession.'

George Teeling Smith sees the uneven-handed use of the skills and resources available as one of medicine's most intractable dilemmas. 'It parallels precisely the North–South world problem. There are underprivileged groups in the world, and in Britain, and in what's called the "underclass" in the USA, and it's extremely difficult.'

He singled out Britain's large immigrant communities as being specially deprived. 'They often don't speak the language, so it's difficult to communicate with them. They're reluctant to learn the language because of ethnic inhibitions. Their understanding of medical and scientific matters is generally extremely poor, and it's difficult to communicate with them. It's very unfair to blame the health service for the fact that social classes four and five smoke many more cigarettes than social classes one and two. That's not a failure of the NHS, but a sociological phenomenon which has to be tackled much more fundamentally.'

He went on to point out that women in social classes four and five don't go to antenatal clinics until much later than women in social classes one and two. 'They read the wrong papers. The *Sun* and *Star* do very little to promote positive health behaviour as compared with the *Guardian* or the *Independent*, which are full of health education articles. People who read the *Sun* or *Star* don't get the benefit of such articles, even if they're able to read English.'

Professor Smith described another fashion in which inequalities of medical care might operate – not from the patients' but from the doctors' side. 'If you ask renal physicians and surgeons whether they are turning away patients, you find that they are not. They actually have the facilities to treat everything that gets to them. But there's a rationing that goes on at the general physician and GP level. They don't say, "I won't refer you for treatment because I know you won't get it." What they're actually saying is, "I don't think you deserve it, in terms of your age or morbidity, or whatever."

'And they're making the right decisions. I sincerely believe that if you've got a seventy-year-old who goes into renal failure the humane decision is to say, "You've achieved just about the average in terms of life expectancy, and I don't think it's right to put you on renal dialysis, bearing in mind the quality of life you'll have for perhaps another five years. You've seen your grandchildren growing up. Your wife is going to have to come to terms with being a widow at some stage, and if she does that without having to visit you in hospital three times a week, or helping you to work the renal dialysis machine for five years, so much the better." I'm taking the moral position that death is more sensible than a survival for three or four or five years which depends on the use of hi-tech medicine.'

However, while all septuagenarians are equal, some, it seems, may be more equal than others. Professor Smith went on to say that while doctors are already rationing medical care implicitly (by, for example, choosing not to book their elderly patients in for a full and expensive 90,000-mile service, and abandoning them instead to a last spluttering journey to the breaker's yard), economists would argue that the basis of such rationing should be a little more explicit, and a little less of a lottery. But then he added, 'That may be wrong. Maybe it's better as a lottery. I know somebody not much younger than you who was very near to renal failure and who very nearly needed a transplant. He actually recovered, but they were quite prepared to look for a kidney in his case. And I think that's right. He was a member of the medical profession, and a highly intelligent person who still had a lot to contribute to the world and to his family. Whereas when it comes to the West Indian who has a miserable pension which is inadequate by any reasonable standards, and who already probably has great-grandchildren because of the fecundity of the race, it's perhaps less serious if he doesn't get the transplant or the dialysis.'

Less serious for what or whom? For the poverty-stricken pater-familial West Indian, or for his wife and sons and daughters, or for the society within which he lives, or for the conscience of the doctor who decides that it's not worthwhile to make an effort to keep the man alive?

Not only do doctors find it easier to deal with their own sort, but they also prefer to work in pleasant places or in centres of excellence where the availability of good medical care already exists.

Barry Salter was a Family Practitioner Committee administrator at the time of our meeting. He served in two districts of Greater London and in North Yorkshire and in Suffolk before going to Cambridge-shire, so he has had a fairly varied experience. Family Health Services Authorities (FHSAs), which have replaced FPCs, are, *inter alia*, responsible for ensuring that adequate general medical services (pretty well everything except hospital-based and public health affairs) are available within their bailiwick. I asked whether he had found much variation in the quality of care provided.

'Yes. Rural counties tend to be able to provide a better standard. You've got space, so it's easier to provide surgeries. They are also, perhaps, more attractive to the more able or more energetic practitioners, who'd like to practise in a nice rural setting. So GPs in pleasant areas have the pick of young doctors who want to enter general practice. Certainly in Croydon and Bromley there were some very able GPs and some very well-run practices. The variations are greater in urban areas, but even in rural areas you do get practices which are not so good.'

What, I suspect, Barry Salter was being too diplomatic to say, is that there are still too many practices which are, by any standards, deplorable, and that the poor practices and places have to make do with the poorer of the new recruits, so that there are self-perpetuating nests and areas of poor primary health care, and that the pleasanter places enjoy the services of the better doctors.

George Teeling Smith comments that 'The best doctors want to practise in Edinburgh or Bournemouth or the better parts of London, and don't want to practise in "Tootington" or up North.' And this inclination applies to hospital medicine as well. 'If you're a registrar with ambitions you don't take a job in Burnley or Southwold. You try to get a job in a teaching hospital in Edinburgh or Glasgow or London. I don't think you can direct doctors to go to underprivileged areas. The distinction between excellence and mediocrity, however undesirable, is extremely difficult to eliminate.'

The new contract for GPs, introduced in April 1990, as the result of the latest Medical Act, may increase the temptation to concentrate upon serving the interests of 'better-class' patients, to the neglect of those who are most in need of medical aid.

GPs will receive a bonus for performing cervical smears on their lady customers aged between twenty-five and sixty-five every five years, and for ensuring that their child customers are up-to-date with their immunizations. But the full bonus will only be paid if 80 per cent of the relevant women on their list, and 90 per cent of the children, have been so served.

It is a worthy idea, presumably dreamed up by civil servants and politicians, and aimed at encouraging GPs to devote more of their energies to the prevention of disease, but it is likely to be counterproductive. Doctors can't (yet) *force* their clients to accept treatment, so GPs are likely to be lukewarm towards customers on their lists of a kind who threaten their incomes. It is well established that people in the lower social groups have a poor record of seeking preventive, as opposed to curative, medical care for themselves and their children, so any practice whose list includes a substantial proportion of underprivileged families will have difficulty in fulfilling its quota of prophylactic measures.

Early last year Community Health Councils throughout the country reported that growing numbers of patients were being removed from doctors' lists (GPs have a right to rid themselves of unwanted customers without necessarily stating a reason), and the CHCs suspected that many of the removals were financially inspired. In April 1990 three doctors in group practice near Carlisle caused a minor furore when they announced that they would not accept patients from two run-down council estates within their area, and said that they might boycott other patients who refused to cooperate in their screening and inoculation programmes. They stated frankly that these moves were aimed at preventing the loss of 'large sums of money'.

It is, of course, possible that this was a clever propaganda exercise, designed to highlight a widely shared criticism of the relevant clauses in the new contract, but there is now an obvious and powerful incentive for GPs to spurn customers who may damage their 'business'.

The new contract also allows practices above a certain size to apply to become budget holders, whereby they will be allocated an annual sum, calculated on the size of their lists, to be used at the members' discretion for the care of their clients, including the 'purchase' of hospital and other services. The theory is that this will increase GP and patient choice, and stimulate hospitals and other agencies to provide efficient service at an attractive and competitive price. Many fear, however, that budgets will make patients with chronic and costly-to-treat diseases an unwelcome burden on the practice funds.

Certainly the new arrangements seem likely to accentuate rather than diminish existing inequalities in medical care, and to provide new and additional reasons for GPs to dispense their services with an uneven hand.

The Government has made an effort to improve the medical services in poorly doctored areas by offering cash incentives (possibly up to £10,000 a year) to GPs (not hospital doctors) willing to work in unattractive places and take on 'difficult' customers, and I asked George Teeling Smith whether you could, indeed, bribe doctors into taking on tough parishes. He had no doubts in the matter.

'No. The middle-class ethic is that you don't line your pocket today against the chance of success in the future. It's no good offering a Junior Hospital Doctor 50 per cent plus to go to Burnley. He's still going to take 50 per cent less to remain with the elite of his profession in London.'

All this agonizing about the inequitable distribution of the 'best doctors' begs the question of how you define such animals. Anybody on the Medical Register can put up a plate wherever he may choose and wait (or, these days, advertise) for custom. I could do that tomorrow, and doubtless supplement my old age pension and meagre literary earnings by several thousand pounds a year with small effort, particularly if I let it be known that I was keen on homoeopathy, or crystal therapy, or the laying on of hands, or some similarly mystical approach to healing. It is only when you want to obtain a contract to service patients on behalf of the NHS that you have to obtain the approval of the local FHSA. The 'best doctors' are not necessarily the most highly qualified or most expert or most knowledgeable or most ambitious or most intelligent and articulate members of the medical profession. The best doctors are those who by temperament and experience are best suited to serve their patients' needs, and a Bangladeshi GP in Bradford may well be just as valuable a member of the medical tribe as, say, Sir Roy Calne, beavering away at his liver transplants in Cambridge.

All this apart, it has to be admitted that poor places tend to be served by poor practitioners. The only encouraging aspect of the situation is that its existence is widely recognized and deplored. There is a scattering of 'missionaries' who go out of their way to help the underprivileged, such as a group of volunteer doctors who run a weekly clinic from an ambulance for London's 'Cardboard City' homeless, and Dr Mary Hepburn, a consultant at Glasgow Royal Maternity Hospital, who has successfully persuaded many of the district's 'outcast' women – drug users, prostitutes, AIDS sufferers, and the like – to use her department's services by making them feel cared for, avoiding moralistic and censorious attitudes, and organizing clinics and advice sessions in a manner that fits in as easily as possible with the customers' often burdensome and ill-structured daily lives. However, Professor Bosanquet has predicted that in five to ten years' time there will be an even greater difference in the standards of service offered to the blessed and to the unblessed.

Ellis Downes, the young house officer, still an idealist, is acutely aware of the fact that certain categories of patient, such as the mentally disabled, get a raw deal compared to the clients of specialists working in more fashionable and prestigious fields like neurology and cardiology. He would like the profession to sort out its priorities in a manner that distributed effort and resources to the best advantage of the nation's health and happiness. But he is impatient with the concept of an ill-served 'underclass', claiming that the State has a duty to *force* its citizens to take responsibility for their own health. 'In America you can't put your children into primary school unless they've been vaccinated, so in the USA you've got the lowest incidence of measles in the world.' He suggests that the same rule should apply here in respect of the principal vaccinations, and believes we might go further. 'You might even say that you can only get your Family Allowance if, when you register, you can show that you've had the required medical servicing during the previous three years.'

I can well remember voicing similar sentiments in the Junior Hospital Doctors' mess when I was his age. We were then, half a century ago, equally irritated by the apparently wilful and obstinate refusal of the *hoi polloi* to conduct their lives in the manner which we had been brought up to regard as proper and responsible.

You can't make people healthy by decree. It's up to governments and doctors and all other labourers in the health vineyard to arrange matters so that the best of health care is readily available to all, and in a fashion that encourages citizens to use the benefits on offer of their own free will.

The Patients' Voice

Although the ideal doctor–patient relationship is one of partnership, it still, too often, appears to be an 'us versus them' affair. Indeed, Dr Joe Collier has recently written a book entitled *The Health Conspiracy* in which he argues his belief that the Government, the medical profession and the pharmaceutical industry attempt and connive (perhaps not even consciously) to manipulate both the provision of medical services and also the citizens in need of health care in a manner which best serves the providers' own interests rather than those of the customers whose needs should be sovereign.

I asked Dr Collier whether *Health Cock-up* might not have been a more appropriate if less elegant title for a book which examines the circumstances under which the consumers of medical care often seem to get less than a fair deal.

'If you are a patient in social class five and go to the doctor, he won't listen to you but will give you some drugs. If you ask questions he'll say, "Don't bother me – take your medicine – go away – don't be impertinent." If you want a second opinion you won't get one. If you're in that position you're right to feel that the medical Establishment is against you. And it conspires against you every way you turn. You don't get communicated with. You see them as alien. They give you the wrong medicines without thinking about things. You try and find out what went wrong and you can't. You try to get another doctor and you can't. You get a lawyer on your side and he can't get the notes. If he does get the notes it costs a lot of money, and it takes years to sort things out. And if you happen to be a white middle-class male it's just as bad. If you want to find out where things went wrong, you won't, except with a tremendous amount of expense and time.

'That isn't a cock-up. That is medicine saying, "I have my own interests, and I protect them, and you can keep away, thank you, because we don't want to be challenged."'

Dr Collier doesn't deny that cock-ups contribute to poor relationships between doctors and their patients, but firmly maintains that the outsider, and with good reason, perceives the system as an opponent. Others, like Rabbi Neuberger, believe that lack of mutual understanding and poor communication, rather than any essential conflict of interests, account for the difficulties which exist.

Whoever is right, the profession is now under challenge from its customers, and this, apart from a few poisoned darts launched by writers like Molière and Shaw, is a fairly recent phenomenon, and one encouraged by the launching of the NHS.

There are now a growing number of organizations devoted to the protection and advancement of patients' interests, and this wouldn't have happened unless there had been a pretty strong feeling for the need.

One of the first of these was the Patients Association, founded in 1963. Julia Neuberger is the present Chairman of the Association which has only around 1,000 members and a small permanent staff, but wields an influence wholly disproportionate to its size.

A telephone advisory service is well used by numerous citizens who have no connection with the Association, but who are led to seek help by CHCs, or by their own doctors, or after reference to one of the health directories now published in an attempt to help the punters find their way around the health care jungle. The Association doesn't pursue complaints on behalf of enquirers, but tells them how to go about the task. Supplicants are often referred to one of the now numerous special interest groups which deal with the needs of sufferers from particular ailments, like multiple sclerosis or deafness or blindness or mental disability, or arthritis, or cystic fibrosis.

The PA is cooperating with other like-minded organizations in attempts to identify the major causes of patient discontent. An important source of concern are people with multiple medical and social problems who have difficulty in dealing with the different experts and advisors involved in their care, which creates confusion giving rise to huge distress.

A second major complaint is the difficulty patients experience when they feel they've had a raw deal. 'Most of the people we talk to don't want financial compensation. They want an apology,' says Julia Neuberger. 'But one of the most difficult things to get from a doctor is an apology, because it's considered by the defence societies (the organizations insuring doctors against claims of malpractice) as an admission of liability. That's crazy. It's hard to imagine anything more dotty.'

It seems to me significant that the Association should have survived at all, let alone thrived, because it deals with faults in the behaviour of the medical profession which should not have occurred in the first place. If doctors were properly attuned to their responsibilities and function, and if the NHS was organized and managed in a more 'customer-friendly' fashion, a patients' association would be redundant.

Somewhat more tardily, officialdom recognized the need for giving consumers a voice in their affairs. In 1974 a Labour Government, with the ebullient Barbara Castle in charge of health, established a network of Community Health Councils, designed to act as a loud and influential *vox populi* in the running of NHS affairs. These bodies have (just about) survived the Thatcher revolution.

The scheme is that every health district (the smallest of the administrative divisions of the NHS) should have its own CHC. The Councils normally have eighteen to twenty-four members of whom half are nominated by local authorities, one-third by voluntary organizations devoted to various aspects of health care, such as Mencap and Age Concern, and one-sixth by the Regional Health Authority (the bosses who can decide to do or not do whatever may be asked for).

CHCs, which have a paid secretariat who are employees of the NHS, are expected to give comfort and advice to citizens who have encountered trouble in their dealings with the service. The Councils don't investigate individual complaints but, like the Patients Association, they do tell dissatisfied customers how to seek redress, and, if necessary, act as a 'plaintiff's friend' in complaint procedures, perhaps helping to draft written depositions, or accompanying supplicants to what can be daunting official hearings.

They are also entitled to be consulted on any proposed changes in the pattern of local health services (such as the closing or opening of hospitals and clinics), and have a limited right to visit and report upon NHS institutions within their parish (but not, strangely, GPs' surgeries, which, arguably, are the most important centres of health care).

In principle, CHCs ought to be powerful agencies and the chief means by which the customers of health care can influence the manner in which they are served, but too often they seem to be largely ignored by the medical and administrative functionaries whose performance they are supposed to monitor.

Margaret Martin wants the CHCs to have broader powers and sharper teeth. 'The way we're doing it now won't work in the future. Every CHC has got to face that, and some don't like it. They want to go on in their little old pompous way, just dealing with complaints, and not addressing wider issues. But most of us now recognize that we've got to put up a different model.'

She finds that doctors are shocked and embarrassed to discover that their customers can become angry and emotional when discontented and confused by the treatment they receive, because 'that's not the British way'. (Well, it's not the way of the sort of Britons who become doctors, and know all about the central value of stiff upper lips.)

Margaret Martin lectures to medical students at Addenbrookes Hospital in Cambridge, and finds that they are absolutely convinced that even admitting their mistakes will lower their status. They don't realize that all most of the complainants who come to her office want is that doctors should concede that they are human, like the rest of us, and that they can make mistakes, and are willing to learn from their errors.

Ellis Downes takes a somewhat different view. He believes that only doctors should regulate the provision of medical services because 'in the end only doctors know about disease. They're trained in recognizing, treating and preventing disease. The Government role in setting up CHCs has been a token effort, to be seen to be giving the public a voice. But they're recognized by most people to be pretty inefficient. They've produced some good reports, but have been clouded by left-wing bias.'

Ay, there's the rub. The profession still instinctively resents anybody outside the club who may attempt to tell doctors how to manage their affairs, and, in a knee-jerk response, tends to regard those who do as 'lefties', except of course when, as now, they happen to be 'righties'. (Incidentally, Margaret Martin has found that a marked change of attitude toward CHCs has occurred among GPs since the Government embarked upon the latest NHS reforms. Family doctors, clearly seeing the patients' representative as a useful ally in the battle against a common foe, now contact her Council, and attend meetings, and take an active part in discussions, and invite Council members to their own meetings, in a way that hadn't happened before.

In Cambridge most of Margaret Martin's time is taken up with dealing with individuals who feel they have a grudge against the NHS, or who just can't cope with the complexities of the service, and, like Julia Neuberger, she finds that most of the complainants would be satisfied with an explanation or, if appropriate, an apology, and don't want money.

Litigation

The fact that most of the patients who complain about some aspect of their dealings with doctors are not seeking a cash balm for their real or imagined wounds may not be perceived by the public at large, because all the publicity goes to the very small minority of dissatisfied customers who do adopt the costly, lengthy and frustrating course of seeking legal redress, and who finally win their case. In recent years British courts have been awarding huge sums in damages to people, or to the relatives of people, who have suffered death or grievous bodily harm as a result of medical mistakes and accidents, so we are beginning to ape a relatively new and destructive legal assault upon doctors (who, inevitably, sometimes perform with less than perfect skill and judgment), of a kind that has become commonplace in the USA.

This profitable exploitation of the mistakes of one profession by another has reached absurd proportions in North America because lawyers in that land of the free are allowed to take on cases on a 'No Win, No Fee' basis, whereby advocates can represent litigants in the courts on the understanding that there's no charge for their services, but that they will receive a healthy cut of any damages won.

This, of course, means that lawyers seek out damaged or less than satisfied customers of the medical profession and *encourage* them to sue. It can reach absurd lengths, as when, recently, an American woman sued her friendly neighbourhood shrink because, she claimed, he had failed to prevent her from going entirely round the twist and murdering her child.

The result of this quite wicked pursuit of money rather than justice by American lawyers is that premiums for professional liability insurance in the USA are now so swingeing that doctors are avoiding high-risk specialties (notably obstetrics), which are the most costly to protect, so that the pattern of practice is distorted in a manner that fails to reflect patient need. And, of course, the cost of care goes up to the benefit of lawyers, and not doctors, and certainly not patients, except for the few who happen to hit the jackpot when playing the medical accident fruit machine.

The threat of litigation has also encouraged the growth of so-called 'defensive medicine' in the USA. This means that doctors' customers are frequently subjected to a whole range of unnecessary and costly and potentially harmful investigations and treatments (like x-rays) simply to avoid any future charge that the doctor hasn't done a proper job (although this factor has only accentuated an already strong, not to say scandalous, habit of excessive medical intervention in a country where doctors are generally rewarded on a fee-per-item-of-service basis).

It's beginning to happen here too. So far we've largely avoided making superfluous treatment profitable, although the new GP contracts and the 'internal market' system being imposed upon the hospital services may prove to have been a step towards such a pernicious state of affairs. But the lawyers (including the judges) may have preempted the politicians in the move towards making medicine a business rather than an art and a science and a calling. This is bad for the consumer, and should be stamped upon. Luckily for both doctors and their customers British lawyers aren't yet permitted to work on a 'No Win, No Fee' contract, although the desirability of such an arrangement has been floated from barristers' chambers within recent months.

What *has* happened is that Britain's medical defence societies have begun to copy their American counterparts by considering widely different premiums for different kinds of doctors, with, once again, obstetricians riding high on the list of 'bad risks'.

There are two moves that ought to be made in order to avoid the shape and nature of medical practice and attitudes becoming distorted by fear of the power of the courts.

The first, and simplest, is the adoption of a 'no fault' compensation policy, whereby the victims of medical mishaps (including the unexpected side-effects of drugs) would have their consequential financial needs met from central funds. This quite tiny drain on the national wealth could, if necessary, be well paid for by a minuscule extra tax on the healthy profits of the pharmaceutical industry, or even on the price of petrol or the profits of the oil conglomerates (motoring, upon which the oil companies depend for most of their income, is, after all, a major cause of cost to the NHS), or perhaps on alcohol and tobacco, which also cost the service dear. And such an arrangement would by no means prevent the truly negligent from being sued (perhaps by the Government instead of the individual) for the cost of their neglect.

The second, and perhaps more difficult to achieve, is for doctors and health authorities to become much more open and understanding in their dealings with their clients, so that mistakes are readily acknowledged (doctors and managers know very well when they've slipped up – who better?), and a gracious admission of fault, or, in the absence of fault, a patient explanation of what went wrong and why, defuses anger and discontent, and reduces the growth of costly formal enquiries and litigation.

As Margaret Martin wisely remarks, it's all about partnership. In a good health service the providers and consumers of medical care must be colleagues, and not opponents on the opposite sides of a fence.

Meanwhile, the situation has ensured the rapid rise to prominence of one of the newer recruits to the growing band of voluntary organizations dedicated to championing the patients' cause. Action for the Victims of Medical Accidents gives free advice and puts complainants in touch with a solicitor who specializes in cases of medical negligence. We shall be justified in feeling satisfied with the manner in which NHS managers and doctors handle their customers only when AVMA finds itself with not enough to do, and decides to go out of business.

5 Regulating Doctors

Doctors are proud and jealous of their status as members of a self-regulating profession. The strongly hierarchical nature of the trade has been a major means by which self-regulation has been sustained. The princes of the healing guild define required patterns of training and activity and behaviour, which have then been imposed upon the medical *hoi polloi* by a system of sanctions. Ethical and social pressures filter down through the chains of command, and the patronage upon which junior club members depend for their advancement in the game is used to discourage dissent. The profession has been an oligarchy, largely immune to external influence.

Things are changing. The rank and file are demanding ever more say in the manner in which their professional lives are arranged, and outsiders, from politicians to individual consumers of health care, are making their voices heard, and developing the clout needed to ensure that their criticisms and requirements are observed.

Some three decades ago Lord Moran, Winston Churchill's physician, who gained notoriety when he published intimate details of his illustrious patient's physical misfortunes, described GPs to a Royal Commission on doctors' pay as unfortunates who had 'fallen off the ladder' of professional achievement.

This was, and is, pernicious nonsense, and today not even the most insensitive and self-satisfied of medical moguls would dare to voice such sentiments abroad. Lord Moran's patronizing view of family medicine is still slightly held in secret by many a clever hospital doctor, but the more discerning members of the profession, and informed observers and administrators of the system, now acknowledge that a high proportion of the brightest and most energetic of new medical graduates are choosing to work in the

community, and that a strong corps of well-trained general practitioners, backed by adequate resources in the way of premises,
technical aids (computers, diagnostic machines and similar tools),
and, most importantly, a staff skilled in such matters as administration, general and specialized nursing techniques, and counselling,
will become the principal means of delivering good medical care in
the years ahead. Lord Moran's 'drop-outs' look set to become
medicine's top dogs.

Way back in the Middle Ages there were three distinct branches of
the healing trade. At the top of the pyramid sat the physicians –
scholars and gentlemen who had received a doctorate in physic from
one of Europe's ancient universities (usually Oxford or Cambridge),
and who dealt with the maladies of the nobs. Next came the barber–
surgeons, who, in addition to cutting their clients' hair and trimming
their beards, would, when the occasion so demanded, let blood, or
cut for the stone, and perform similar manipulations of the flesh.
Finally, at the bottom of the pile, were the apothecaries, who made
their living by dispensing the remedies prescribed by their betters,
the physicians, and who also acted as the people's therapists.

There was bitter rivalry between the three castes, each wanting to
maximize its share of the profit to be made from disease. But a kind
of unity was finally imposed upon the different groups by the
Medical Act of 1858. Thereafter, all who aspired to the title
'doctor', in the medical sense, and a place on the newly created
Medical Register, had to undergo a prescribed course of training,
and to pass a series of standardized examinations.

Thus, in theory, all doctors have been born equal since 1858. But,
as is very well known, laws can't change tribal attitudes and
customs, and the old divisions long and until only very recently
remained, with physicians heading the hierarchy, surgeons running
a close second, and GPs (the old apothecaries) coming a poor third,
the only difference being that the sorting-out process began after
qualification, and not before admission to the guild.

For a time the Act of 1858 did have a levelling-out effect, for all
those admitted by examination to the Medical Register were deemed
competent to practise medicine, surgery and midwifery, and their
training was designed to fit them for the role, and they largely took
advantage of the fact.

Thus, in the century preceding World War II, there was no essential difference between the clinical activities of 'hospital doctors' and 'family doctors'. Most GPs were sturdy all-rounders performing nearly all the tasks which are now the preserve of specialists. Every family doctor was accustomed to cutting out an inflamed appendix, perhaps, with luck, in the local cottage hospital, or sometimes on the customer's kitchen table, and was adept at delivering babies. He would also take full charge of the victims of heart disease, diabetes, pneumonia, syphilis, anaemia and many another condition of a kind nowadays automatically regarded as demanding specialist attention. The Jack-of-all-trades nature of the family doctor's daily round was as much a matter of necessity as choice, for when World War II broke out there *were* only some 3,000 consultants in the UK, compared to 20,000-plus GPs.

The 'consultants' in places like Shrewsbury or Coventry or Watford were essentially GPs who had gained a local reputation for their special interest in dealing with gall-bladder disease or broken hips or whatever, and who had got themselves appointed as honorary members of the medical staff of their local voluntary hospitals. At a 'higher' level consultants were drawn from among the more thrusting and ambitious new graduates, who remained at their teaching hospitals, unpaid or on a subsistence wage, as the dogsbodies of their chiefs on the honorary staff. During this postgraduate apprenticeship they would take a higher qualification offered by one of the Royal Colleges – the FRCS if they wanted to be surgeons, or the MRCP if they aimed to become physicians. Both these badges of special competence have to be earned by the passing of stiff and (in effect) competitive examinations in which the casualty rate is high, and a first-time pass is counted a considerable achievement.

After ten or fifteen years of such gruelling vassalage, the neophyte might hope to become an honorary consultant himself. (The same system operates today, except that the so-called Junior Hospital Doctors and their bosses are now well paid by Mother State.) This is the 'ladder' which Moran accused GPs of having fallen off.

The chiefs were called 'honoraries' because that's exactly what they were, doing their work at the great voluntary hospitals for nothing, or for a token stipend of maybe £50 a year. They filled their beds with the sick poor who were 'fortunate' enough to suffer from some sufficiently interesting malady, or whose state made them 'good teaching material'. They made their living exclusively from private patients whom they saw in their consulting rooms in places like Harley Street, or who were treated at home, or in nursing homes, or in the private wings of the consultants' hospitals. These hospitals were their power base, and the places where they made their reputations, and their charity work was essential to their worldly success. They remained comparatively few in number because only the larger towns and cities sustained major voluntary hospitals and (just as importantly) a rich reservoir of prospective paying customers.

However, the humble GPs began to resent the competition for well-heeled clients presented by the hospital glamour boys with their subtly advertised expertise. The threat of a really ugly internecine feud grew large, but this, in the end, could only have harmed business and damaged medicine's brand image, which, before the days of effective drugs, was one of the doctors' principal therapeutic weapons. So, something like a century ago, the commonality of doctors, represented by the youthful British Medical Association (founded in 1832, and originally called the Provincial Medical and Surgical Association), came to an agreement with the then existing Royal Colleges (others have sprouted since), which were the consultants' guilds.

The bargain was that the physicians and surgeons who set themselves up as specialists would not see any private patients except at the request of the customer's own personal or family practitioner. The 'provincial' or 'village' or 'high street' doctors now felt secure, and were happy to send some of their more puzzling patients (those who could manage the fee) to a consultant colleague for a second opinion. (Hence the title 'consultant', which is not found abroad.)

Family doctors still went on doing anything they felt to be within their competence (and maybe a good deal else besides), and not many people ever did see a specialist. But since the patricians were fairly thin on the ground, they did well enough out of the deal. Instead of having to attract their own patients, they were able to sit back and await the arrival of those referred by their ex-pupils, or by local practitioners who knew of their fame. Everybody was more or less happy.

This arrangement survived the coming of the NHS, and is the basis of the present British rule whereby hospital consultants can only be approached through the good offices of your friendly neighbourhood GP. The rule has nothing to do with any rational idea that these experts ought to be protected from clients whose needs don't demand their peculiar skills, although it does happen to be a convenient tradition for a State medical service. It is a trade convention, which does not apply in the rest of the Western world, including the USA, where its absence does no noticeable detriment to the health of the inhabitants. Its existence severely limits the customer's freedom of choice, and perhaps it should be proscribed as a restrictive trade practice. The original agreement became the final bar in the gate dividing the profession.

After the end of World War II Britain's Labour Government and its dedicated Health Minister, Aneurin Bevan, were determined to fulfil their election pledges and achieve an admirable aim by launching a National Health Service, providing full medical care, free to all at the time of need, and to do so with the least possible delay. This is why the existing structure, which was the result of 'happenstance' and history, and not the consequence of any kind of intelligent planning, was taken over wholesale by the State. In adopting this easy option our Lords and Masters fluffed a unique opportunity for setting up a system of medical care which would exploit the skills and resources available in a manner which would best benefit the needs of the nation at the smallest cost. As a result, successive Governments have felt the need to undertake a series of 'reorganizations' which have succeeded in confusing and upsetting everybody concerned without altering the fundamental shape or inborn deficiencies of the beast, and it seems likely that the latest and current package of 'reforms' will have much the same effect.

But despite taking over the medical world 'as found', instead of attempting to devise a model scheme for the delivery of medical care from scratch, Bevan found that enormous problems had to be overcome, the greatest of which was the fierce opposition of the medical profession. Doctors of all kinds, from the most senior and powerful metropolitan specialists to the most humble and unassuming country family practitioners, were determined to maintain their traditional and accustomed way of life, and, in particular, were desperately afraid of any Government interference with their precious independence and 'clinical freedom'. They were scared stiff of becoming civil servants.

In the field of general practice Bevan wanted the health ministry – the paymaster – to control the distribution of family doctors serving the NHS, and to abolish the sale of practices (so that the gift and distribution of medical parishes should belong to the State), and to make family doctors salaried employees of the service. He got away with the first two of these demands, but, with family doctors threatening to refuse to join the scheme, he backed down on the third and allowed GPs to work for the NHS as 'independent contractors'. (See Chapter 7.)

To get the grudging cooperation of the consultants (who had powerful representatives at court, including the great wheeler-dealer, Moran), Bevan had to make a number of concessions. Consultants were to be given a proper professional salary for their work in the nation's hospitals, all of which (save for a special few) would become the health minister's property on 'the appointed day'. However, the senior and already established specialists were determined not to sacrifice their often extremely lucrative private work. Nye Bevan was forced to strike a bargain whereby any consultant could work part-time for the NHS and part-time for himself.

Since then about half have elected to work on the so-called maximum part-time basis, whereby they receive nine-elevenths of the full salary appropriate to their posts in return for a notional nine half-day NHS sessions a week. For the rest of the time they can do their own thing. In effect this means that they can order their affairs pretty much as they choose, so long as the hospital work gets done. Many of the consultants who do opt for full-time employment belong to the less fashionable specialties, such as geriatrics and psychiatry, where the chance of a steady flow of private work is low. (In the USA, of course, many thousands of citizens employ private shrinks, but this is not so far the case in the UK.) Academics (lecturers and professors in the various branches of clinical medicine) are paid by their universities and given honorary NHS appointments, and the income from any private work they undertake goes into their departments' research funds.

In addition to allowing them to continue their profitable extramural activities, the Minister had to agree to the notorious system of merit awards (further discussed below) whereby one-third of the country's consultants now receive a secret additional income in recognition of exceptional worth. This 'sweetener' was wrung out of Bevan by Moran (who else?) on the grounds that some extra inducement was necessary in order to persuade 'good' men to enter and stay with the NHS.

By these means Bevan effectively bought off the consultants' opposition to the new service, and, lacking these powerful allies, the GPs surrendered too, taking what comfort they could from the fact that they had fought off the threat to make them salaried servants of the State. Having tamed the potentates Bevan boasted that he had 'stuffed their mouths with gold'. He is often accused by medical politicians of having divided the profession in order to rule. This is nonsense. He simply took advantage of the fact that the healing trade had already split itself in two, and in a fashion far more effective and complete than any outsider could have imposed.

The creation of the NHS at first diminished the status of the family doctor. The 3,000-strong corps of consultants available at the time the service was born was rapidly augmented, and had increased five-fold by 1988, so that there are now nearly half as many specialists as GPs.

This means that an 'expert' in the handling of eczema, or cystitis, or anxiety, or whatever, became available for consultation no more than a bus ride away from the homes of a majority of the citizens of the land. Lazy or unconfident or incompetent GPs were thus presented with a simple method for offloading clients whose requirements interfered with their golf or profitable sidelines or peace of mind, and their more able, conscientious and industrious colleagues often felt constrained to refer their challenging and interesting cases to the local expert simply in order to ensure that their patrons benefited from the best available advice. Hospital out-patient departments became crowded with patients who would previously have remained the responsibility of their personal physicians.

Even so, there was little true cooperation between the hospital moguls and their High Street brothers. Wendy Savage recalls that when she was a student in the late 1950s the consultants hardly knew the names of the local GPs, and when they did it was only to complain how frightful they were.

'I've never forgotten a doctor with a lock-up shop in Cable Street (a pretty run-down East London thoroughfare). He used to go in for an hour, then all his patients would turn up in casualty with notes on bits of lavatory paper just saying "Please see and treat". One day he sent up a man with cellulitis who had a huge abscess in his forearm which should never have been allowed to develop. Well, enough was enough. The creature was incompetent. Then we discovered that he had a private practice in Harley Street which he went to after his hour's stint for the NHS. So we began to ring him up there every time we saw one of his patients and say, "Thank you so much, doctor, for referring this interesting case – we've done this, this and this." After a week we didn't have another case from him. He sent them all to Poplar.'

She also recalls a note that came with a patient who'd been seen by a doctor who was doing a locum in a similar practice which read, 'I'm sorry for referring this patient to you, but in this surgery there's a desk and a chair and nothing else.'

The offloading of patients needing anything more than the most casual attention and a hastily scribbled prescription meant that a doctor so inclined could indeed fulfil the letter, if not the spirit, of his contract with the NHS, working from the most primitive and ill-equipped of premises. But with a national network of well-equipped and well-staffed hospitals taking over so much routine, let alone specialized, investigation and therapy, even excellent GPs working from well-found surgeries often felt that they had become little more than sorting clerks and pill dispensers. This was certainly a view taken by many medical visitors from abroad, and particularly those from North America, who wondered how it was possible to dream up a system of health care which excludes half its doctors from experiencing the professional satisfaction of dealing with major acute illness, and which removes patients from the care of a familiar and trusted physician at the very time when they are most in need of comfort and support.

In fact the division, involving the apparent near-castration of Moran's medical 'underclass', may prove to have been the salvation of general practice, and a prime cause of its resurgence, even to the extent that family doctors will end up ruling the roost, which happening could at last lead to Britain's NHS truly becoming the 'envy of the world'.

Family or 'community' medicine practically disappeared in many Western countries in the post-war era, with most doctors setting themselves up as mini- or maxi-'specialists' of one kind or another, open to approach from any customer who might fancy sampling the particular brand of therapy they offered. Only in Britain was the pattern of general practitioners, with a list of committed and regular clients, for whom they were the first port of call and the only gateway to the rest of the system, set in legislative concrete. The survival of the caste was assured, because entering general practice was the only way a majority of medical graduates could assure themselves a living.

So while GPs appeared by law established to be condemned to a humble and subsidiary role in the medical scene for ever, what actually happened was that the neutered half of the profession was powerfully inspired to seek a greater role, and an increase in its status.

Nobody expected this to happen. Professor Bosanquet says that the rise in importance of primary care has occurred 'against all the odds and all the predictions. In the 1960s the sociologists were predicting the demise of general practice. It has given medicine in Britain a chance to develop a new kind of relationship with the public, and a new credibility with other professions and health service managers and policy makers.'

In 1952 family doctors established their own academic institution, the College of General Practitioners (later to become another Royal), with the intention of providing themselves with a headquarters, and an instrument for influencing and advancing professional standards in their field, and for lobbying authority, of a kind long enjoyed by the consultant. GPs already had the BMA, which had always been largely their affair, and never a major channel for the promotion of the interests of the top brass, but the Association was and is essentially a trade union, primarily concerned with medical politics and the conditions of service offered to its members, and not so much with the quality of service which its members might offer in return.

The new College had a more closely defined purpose. It wanted general practice to earn the right to be regarded as a specialty in its own right, demanding skills and training and understandings just as 'special', and certainly no less important to the common weal, than those possessed by, say, brain surgeons or cardiologists.

The College has prospered. It has established an examination for membership now taken by about 1,500 candidates each year, and in order to pass the supplicant has to show an understanding of not only clinical affairs, but also the workings of the health service and the social security system, and the psychological and ethical aspects of the doctor–patient relationship, and so on and so on. The College also offers a fellowship, at first gifted to grandees of the caste, but now to be earned by tested and demonstrated excellence.

The College has been only one factor, albeit a major one, in the remarkable improvements which have taken place, and the BMA has played an important role on the political side. Discontent had come close to open rebellion by the early 1960s, and the Association organized the resistance movement. It collected signed letters of resignation from its GP members, and, by the time a Labour Government secured power in 1964, was holding 18,000 of these documents in reserve, ready to pass them on to the Health Department unless a series of major demands were met. David Owen is in no doubt that far from bluffing, many of the signatories were ready to leave the NHS entirely and go it alone, which happening could have made the service unworkable.

As a result of this formidable pressure the then Health Minister, Kenneth Robinson, negotiated a new contract with GPs which earned itself the soubriquet of The Family Doctor Charter. One of its most auspicious features was a generous scheme for a substantial reimbursement of practice expenses, including the costs of improving old and building new premises, and employing ancillary staff. Health centres began to appear, and GPs were given the financial incentive to form group practices in place of the traditional, inefficient, and under-resourced if often beloved single-handed or two-partner affairs. Now more than 80 per cent of general practice units are group concerns attracting the income necessary to the provision of a comprehensive service.

Not only do medical schools now make some attempt (some more than others) to give their students an understanding of the realities of and skills particular to family doctoring, but new (or, indeed, experienced) graduates (after their compulsory hospital intern year, which all medical neophytes are required to serve before achieving full registration) must also undergo a period as a trainee or apprentice in an approved general practice (that is, one which has been inspected and certified as doing a good job) before they can be employed by the NHS as 'principals' in this increasingly important branch of medicine.

The isolation of family doctors from the world of hospital medicine is slowly breaking down as consultants and GPs begin to recognize that they depend upon one another if they are to do the best for themselves and their customers. Postgraduate medical centres are now a part of the physical structure of district general hospitals, and in these places family and hospital doctors meet to exchange views and teach one another. Many family doctors do 'sessions' in their local hospitals in clinics and casualty departments. Consultants are beginning to emerge from the security of their ivory towers and to act as true 'consultants' to their family doctor colleagues instead of simply taking over the care of the GPs' customers.

Wendy Savage is one of the pioneers of this desirable development. 'I'm not the only consultant in Tower Hamlets who goes out to GP practices. One of the paediatricians has been going out for a long time. I started off in 1982, going to three practices once a month.' She sees pregnant women either alone or in company with their family doctor, according to the circumstances, and, in either case, provides expert guidance which the GP can then follow. 'What has happened is that over the years the GPs have become much more confident about doing things and discussing things, like doing an amniocentesis or deciding whether there's a need for ultrasound. They are therefore expanding their skills and keeping up with what's going on in the hospital. Textbooks and even articles come out some time after things have changed, but if we visit the GPs they're really kept up-to-date – they know when we want to change a test or do things in a different way. So they feel more confident about their skills, and the women seem to prefer it.

'We've just started a study designed to discover whether women really do prefer this approach, because it may be that some women do feel deprived at not going to the hospital – that somehow there's a second-rate consultant coming out to the clinics – who knows?'

John Marks offers a different response to the idea of consultants becoming advisors on rather than recipients of patient care. 'I think if you take most consultants away from their toys they're not much better than we are. Therefore they have to be in a hospital with their toys. A pathologist without a lab is no use. A radiologist without an x-ray machine is not a lot of joy. And a surgeon without an operating theatre isn't a lot of good either. Now, a psychiatrist is different. I think there's a place for them in the surgery.'

My own feeling is that Wendy Savage and John Marks have, between them, defined the future role of the consultants. Some sorts, of a kind who depend upon the availability of expensive and special machines and facilities in order to exercise their expertise, should stay in their citadels. But hospital beds should only be occupied by patients who truly need twenty-four-hour-a-day nursing and medical care, and hospital out-patient departments should only be used by citizens in need of investigation or manipulation of a kind that can't be well provided in GPs' surgeries. Wherever possible consultants should help GPs in their work instead of taking it over.

There is a problem here, because, denied much of their clinic-fodder, how would the experts experiment and develop their techniques? I put it to Joe Collier that a lot of people in hospital need not be there, and could just as well, and much more cheaply, be handled by their GPs.

'There's a lot of truth in that. There are a lot of people in there because their circumstances don't allow them to go home.' He went on about that kind of thing, including the suggestion that some patients might be kept in hospital just because they don't get on with their GPs, but, most revealingly, that some are kept in because their bodies and beings are needed for research.

Although one can sense that some hospital doctors still feel that GPs have removed themselves from the cutting edge of medicine, and that, once out in the community, their skills and minds (in a medical sense, at least) tend to become blunted for lack of the stimulus of daily contact with competitive colleagues, everybody I spoke to readily conceded that the standard of general practice has improved out of all recognition, and all, perforce, acknowledge the fact that a high proportion of the ablest graduates now opt for a career in family medicine as a first choice, and certainly not because they have fallen off Moran's ladder.

Why this happens is still a matter of opinion. Ellis Downes and Bill Grove, both youngsters in the trade, who have set their hearts on specialist careers, suspect that their contemporaries who are getting out of hospital medicine are doing so for the negative reason that they don't like the look of it. Bill Grove reported a conversation he'd had with a consultant neurosurgeon approaching retirement. 'I asked him whether he'd go into surgery if he were starting all over again. He said that although he'd enjoyed his career enormously, he'd have to think twice about going into any kind of hospital medicine now. The fun's gone out of it. It wasn't the fun of the job. It wasn't the changing techniques of surgery. It was the amount of administration.'

Even the experienced and iconoclastic Joe Collier answered my question about why more and more bright graduates were opting for general practice by saying, 'There's brightness and brightness, and some people's brightness might be directed towards what's going to be an easier life. So, at the age of twenty-three, they might have the brightness to see that they could have a happier and more fulfilled career in terms of leisure time and family life if they go into general practice. And they are right. And I've seen some very clever students go into general practice. But it's ultimately by default.'

Wendy Savage tells a different tale. 'I teach students about general practice. They start off thinking that general practice has a pretty low status and they end up amazed at how hard GPs work, and enthused about the idea of general practice as a specialty.'

I hope and believe that Wendy Savage is right, and that Ellis Downes and Bill Grove and Joe Collier are wrong, and that Julia Neuberger is right when she says that 'We're going to see GPs largely carrying the NHS.'

I hope and believe that a high proportion of the best and the brightest of our medical graduates are choosing a career in general practice because they recognize that that's where they can best fulfil the ambition that brought them into medicine in the first place, which, in Ra Gillon's simple but explicit term, is to help the sick.

If Moran is following events down here from his place in that Great Royal College in the sky, I hope he has the grace to mount an occasional blush.

Junior Hospital Doctors

The status and function of GPs may have changed very much for the better since the health service began, but the position of the so-called Junior Hospital Doctors remains much the same.

The title JHD is applied to anybody below consultant rank, and encompasses all from the just-qualified tyro to the Senior Registrar, which latter person may have had ten or more years' experience in the trade, and will have achieved a higher qualification, and who, as often as not, will be a better and more with-it doctor than his boss, if only because he's younger, and more energetic, and more ambitious.

Anyway, and broadly speaking, the way the system works is that the lower you are in the hospital hierarchy the less you get paid and the more you have to do, which is, I suppose, a pattern typical of every trade. Here's what one recently qualified healer told me of his day.

'I don't think we do too badly. I get a good six hours' sleep most nights. Except, of course, on Tuesdays and Fridays and some weekends when we're on call. I manage at least one meal a day, and quite often two. I was foolish at first, and didn't eat at all if I was busy. Nobody *tells* you to go and have supper. So in the first two months I lost nearly a stone. But that didn't do me any harm.

'I get them to give me a ring at 7 am. I have a bath. I don't usually have time for coffee. I need to be on the ward by 8. That gives me half an hour before I'm due in the theatre.

'Once on the ward I'll do a quick round of roughly thirty patients. I'll examine the three or four who were operated on the day before. Our man mostly does guts, so a number won't be feeding by mouth. They'll be on intravenous drips. I'll have to look at the lab reports and make sure they're getting the right amounts of this and that, and, if need be, order a change of the mixture in the bottle. Then I must say who can start taking fluids by mouth, or who can try taking more than yesterday – or less. I listen to the sounds of their guts. So long as they've got active, noisy guts, there's no need to worry.

'At 8.30 I belt up to the theatre. I'm normally a bit late, but I change and scrub up and start the main work of the day, which is mostly a matter of hanging on to retractors to keep holes open for other people to operate in. In one of the breaks between cases we'll get a cup of coffee if we're lucky. But the coffee lady is a nutty old harridan. She's very tight with "her" coffee, and turns nasty if she thinks you've asked to be served out of season.

'We've probably finished the list by 2 pm, except for one long day a week, when it may go on until 6 or 8. When the last operation's over I'll have forms to fill in to go down to the lab with specimens. Then I'll have to see that any special instructions about patients reach the ward and are understood. After that I might or might not get to the mess for lunch. The food's very cheap and rather nasty. We pay cash on the nail.

'Perhaps you're left in peace for twenty minutes to enjoy the soggy cabbage and braised heart, and perhaps not – the bleep goes roughly thirty times a day. Then it's back to the ward to sort out the problems they'll certainly have waiting for you. Somebody will have stopped peeing, or started vomiting, or have a fever. You have to decide what's wrong and what to do. Then the new patients start coming in. I have to chat them up, write down their histories, examine them, order any special tests, make sure they haven't any unsuspected troubles like heart failure or diabetes – and if they have, do something about it.

'If it's one of the two days a week on which emergency surgical cases come to my wards there'll be extra calls to casualty. One day last week I handled ten emergency admissions between 2 in the afternoon and 5 next morning. Two of them needed immediate operations. I have to arrange all that – book the theatre, find an anaesthetist, get any necessary tests or x-rays done, perhaps put up a drip or arrange for the right sort of blood to be ready for transfusion. And, of course, I have to assist at the operation.

'Meanwhile, life goes on. If I can sneak ten minutes off I get a cup of tea with the nurses in their own little office off the ward. This is strictly forbidden. We're stealing from the NHS. It's "People's Tea" and "People's Sandwiches" we're using. I should go to the mess, and the nurses to their dining hall. We should pay for our cuppas. But it's a long trip. Five minutes there and five minutes back. And we don't have that much time to waste.

'We always talk shop. It's the only real chance we have to chat about our patients. The people who think they're safeguarding the taxpayer's money by forbidding this kind of orgy are bloody idiots. They simply don't understand what hospitals are all about.

'In the evening I have to sit myself down at the desk in the ward, and stick all the lab reports in the patients' files, and write a progress note for everybody, and write letters to GPs. It takes a hell of a time. Any half-sensible secretary could do most of it just as well, and better.

'And it's my job to talk to the relatives, and tell them what's happening. But a far worse job is talking to dying patients. On the whole the doctors on this unit don't tell dying patients the truth. If your boss has said something vague or comforting, even if he knows a person's going to die, you can't just go along later and contradict him. That would raise dreadful torturing doubts. Sometimes I do tell a mortally ill patient what to expect. I do it quickly before anybody else has had a chance to tell a different story. And then I tell my bosses what I've said. But you should be able to spend a proper time on this sort of talk. For God's sake – isn't a dying person at least entitled to half an hour of his doctor's time each day? But I can't find it for them. In any case, this ought to be the consultant's task. *He's* the chap who's supposed to have the experience and understanding. *He's* the chap who can best inspire confidence. And will he do it? Will he hell!

'After supper the rest of the evening is taken up in dealing with problems of patients already on the wards. That's on a quiet day. On a take-in day, of course, anything might happen. I've usually finished by midnight, or 1 or 2 o'clock. So then I go for a last round on the wards, and I drink another stolen mug of NHS tea or Ovaltine or Nescafé with the nurses. And then I put my bleep to bed in its recharging chamber, and then I go to bed myself.

'The telephone might ring a couple of times in the night. If we're not on take-in the calls will be about patients I know, lying in the wards, and perhaps I can answer a nurse's query and go straight back to sleep. But on a Tuesday and Friday and alternate weekends the call will like as not take me down to casualty, and then to the ward, and then to the theatre.

'Officially we do get every other evening off, and every other weekend, and one half day a week. It doesn't work out like that, of course.

'The nastiest time comes just when you're turning in. You've parked your bleep, and you go along for a crap, and you're squatting there, and suddenly you hear a telephone ringing in one of the rooms. And you're convinced it's yours. And there's nothing you can do about it. That really is unpleasant.'

Why do highly intelligent and long-educated young professionals put up with the kind of slavery that would send your average dustman or bank clerk screaming to the European Court of Human Rights?

I think there are several explanations, and that the first amongst these is that they actually enjoy the experience – they find that being 'needed' twenty-four hours a day is an enormous boost to their self-esteem, and that in their vigorous youth they are willing to pay the price for a stimulating drug. (No other profession provides neophytes with such an exciting introduction to the trade. Young barristers aren't stretched to the limit of their ability the moment that they qualify. They become depressed, shuffling papers and waiting for a brief. I don't know what happens to young curates, but I suspect that they, also, flounder around for several years, striving to find a role. That doesn't happen with young doctors. They're in at the deep end from the word 'Go'.) However, the stimulus of suddenly being wanted after six years as a student, and knowing yourself regarded as the lowest form of medical life and a bit of a nuisance to all concerned, won't counteract the stress of unending onerous work forever. 'Apart from the fact that I don't have a social life,' said a young lady obstetrical house officer at the London Hospital recently, 'I'm permanently tired and I have permanent nightmares that I'm in an antenatal clinic and I have failed to spot a very growth-retarded baby. The worst part is when somebody comes in bleeding and terrified and my main thought is "Oh God, I just want to go to bed."'

A second proposition is that JHDs accept their slave status

because they depend upon the good opinion of their chiefs for any hope of advancement in the trade, and are thus subservient and compliant and unwilling to protest.

A third likelihood is that the system is so huge that any attempt to shift it in any direction requires more power and energy than is to hand.

Fourth, managers (whose main preoccupation these days is the saving of money, and whose own income is tied to their success in this worthy but negative activity) have a positive incentive to maintain the status quo because of the extraordinary manner in which JHDs' pay packets are worked out. If you happen to work for British Rail, or Telecom, or any of many other service industries, and you have to do a job on a Sunday, or at night, or after you should have gone home at 'tea-time', or at any other 'anti-social' hour, you get paid well above the 'standard rate'. If you happen to work as a Junior Hospital Doctor for the NHS, then after forty hours your hourly reward (for overtime) is cut by about 60 per cent, so that it well pays hospital administrators to keep tired junior doctors on the job instead of bringing in extra staff. The longer you work, the less you cost.

But perhaps the most depressing aspect of this exploitation of the energy and enthusiasm of the young is that some of the old boys of the trade, and some of the politicians who 'employ' them, don't even recognize that it's happening. Hence David Mellor's famous gaffe in December 1988 when, as Minister of State for Health, he stated his belief that some of the hairier reported examples of errors committed by exhausted Junior Hospital Doctors were 'fishermen's stories'. He was promptly invited by several of the 'fishermen' to spend a few days dogging their footsteps so that he could see for himself what life in the trenches is really like – an opportunity for enlightenment which he strangely failed to accept.

The troops have mutinied, or, rather, made increasingly mutinous noises of a kind that would have been inconceivable when I was a lad. The Junior Hospital Staff Committee of the BMA, working through the 'proper channels', has been pressing for a maximum seventy-two-hour week (gosh! Only seventy-two hours! What's modern youth coming to?), and for JHDs to be paid for overtime at the basic rate at least. In the face of sustained pressure and a steady flow of 'fishermen's stories' (including not a few which have been told in courts of law when patients have sued because of damage suffered under the ministrations of asleep-on-their-feet young agents of the NHS) the Government acknowledged that there *might* be a problem, and undertook to 'do something about it'.

The 'doing something', to be effective, would include the rapid appointment of more consultants so that JHDs were left with a smaller proportion of the clinical load to handle, and of more juniors, and of more secretaries and so forth so that the juniors were relieved of more of their non-medical chores, and proper payments for overtime so that the temptation to use JHDs as cheap labour was removed. But all that kind of thing costs quite a lot of money, so, of course, it hasn't happened. The politicians claim that matters are improving. The JHDs (who should know) claim that they are much the same. This has provoked placard-decorated demonstrations at hospital gates by white-coated youngsters who ought, instead, to be in bed (or at least in the local pub), and in June 1990 they were considering strike action unless their demands were met by Christmas. JHDs did withdraw their labour (or got pretty selective about the kind of labour they'd supply) in the mid-1970s, and, as a result, won the wonderful concession that they would be paid at least something for their overtime. On that occasion patients didn't suffer too much because, in a rare demonstration of solidarity, the consultants agreed to cover for their junior colleagues.

My own view is that most doctors hate strike action, because it abnegates their *raison d'être*, which is to help people, and that any system of control which forces them to such distasteful action must be seriously flawed, and utterly lacking in an understanding of their professional attitudes and purpose.

There are two other major faults in the present pyramid of hospital doctors whereby you have one consultant served by, say, half-a-dozen JHDs. The first is that only one of that half-dozen can hope to take that consultant's (or another's) place when he eventually retires or gets run over by a bus, so that there are many more prospective specialists than there are posts to be had. There is no assured career structure for young hopefuls who opt for the hospital life. Many find, after years of effort, that they have to seek a living elsewhere. Perhaps in general practice, or perhaps abroad somewhere. So there are a lot of frustrated 'senior' Junior Hospital Doctors around.

The second fault is more serious (if you accept the proposition that the NHS is there for the benefit of the patient rather than of the medical profession). There are not enough consultants (that is to say, experienced elders in the medical trade) to ensure the proper training and supervision of their younger colleagues.

A report published in the *British Medical Journal* in 1990 claimed that most of the serious accidents occurring during childbirth could be blamed upon Junior Hospital Doctors who are inadequately supervised and poorly trained, and who might be given advice over the telephone by consultants who should, instead, have been there in the labour ward.

Again in 1990 the Royal College of Surgeons commented on an enquiry which had concluded that up to 1,000 deaths each year occurring during or shortly after surgery were preventable, and had happened because of junior staff carrying out operations outside 'normal hours' without seeking advice from consultants, and the College recommended that consultants should take a greater responsibility for the supervision of trainees.

But is that advice realistic? Wendy Savage says that 'Junior doctors are poorly supervised because a consultant can't supervise three people and see new patients himself. If the consultant was actually sitting with the trainees and teaching them for a time, and didn't have so many trainees that he couldn't supervise them, you could ensure that they were properly taught.'

So there we go again. Lack of sufficient money to appoint a sufficiency of consultants is both hobbling the prospects of Junior Hospital Doctors and damaging their education. More consultants *are* being appointed, but at a painfully slow rate and in an uneven fashion, and, all too often, the immense pressures put upon managers to balance inadequate budgets leads to vacancies caused by death or retirement or resignation to remain unfilled. There is also one gloomy school of thought which holds that, because of inadequate managerial control, any additional consultant posts created don't result in existing units shedding some of their load, but simply lead to more work being taken on.

Perhaps the cynics *are* right when they claim that general practice is attracting refugees rather than disciples.

Top Dogs

Consultants have a vested interest in limiting their own numbers and maintaining the pyramidal shape of the hospital hierarchy. In the first place, as leaders of their own small teams of what amount to personal assistants they enjoy a delicious sense of individual power, and as a relatively small elite they share a real corporate power, giving them an added individual importance which would be diluted if there were too many of them. Would curates accord bishops the fawning respect they now command if there was one in every parish?

Second, if the number of consultants and JHDs were brought nearer to parity, as has been urged, in order to give specialists in training a reasonable chance of achieving top rank, the consultants would clearly have to share more of the chores of daily medicine, otherwise these wouldn't get done.

Third, more consultants would mean that each would control a smaller share of finite resources, or have a smaller chance of nabbing an extra large slice of the NHS cake (as some, such as our more eminent transplanters, do now), or of collaring one of those desirable merit awards. And competition for a share of the highly lucrative private market would increase.

In public the consultants' guilds support the idea of more posts for their kind, but there must be the suspicion that some of the slowness in bringing this about is due to a lack of real determination on the part of the existing incumbents to make it happen.

A fairly recent development has been a system devised by the Royal Colleges whereby recognition of specialist status requires that the candidate must have held a series of approved training posts. These are limited in number, since, to get the royal blessing, a job must provide both experience of high-calibre clinical practice and exposure to superior tutelage, so many a highly competent trainee has his progress blocked simply because he fails in the always fierce competition for such appointments. It is clearly a 'good thing' that the Colleges should endeavour to ensure that those admitted to their specialist registers should not only have demonstrated expert skills and knowledge at a professional examination, but also have served a good apprenticeship. But does the new requirement reflect a pure and altruistic concern for the quality of specialist practice and the welfare of the customers, or might there be an element of protectionism in the scheme, or at least evidence of a determination by the moguls to keep their subordinates thoroughly well in line?

Wendy Savage comments that 'Younger doctors are even more aware than their older colleagues of the need for a patron, and of keeping your nose clean, and not opening your mouth and rocking the boat. In the past there was enough flexibility in the system to allow mavericks like me to do their own thing and still end up in a position of some influence. But now, with all these career requirements, it's becoming so sewn up that I think we may see a decline.'

But achieving a prized consultancy by no means frees the ambitious younger hospital doctor from domination by his elders and betters. Those blessed merit awards are among a number of factors which see to that.

Some 200 grandees of the profession hold so-called A-plus awards which double their considerable basic salaries. About 4,000 hold C awards, worth roughly one-fifth of the glittering top prize. In between, some 700 and 1,700 hold A and B awards respectively, worth intermediate amounts.

About 60 per cent of all consultants will have won some kind of award by the time they retire, the top earners having worked their way up through the ranks. Broadly speaking, C awards go to those who have achieved a local reputation, Bs go to the nationally known, A awards to outstanding performers with an international reputation, and A-pluses to gurus like the presidents of the Royal Colleges and their cronies in the higher councils of the trade.

In theory every consultant is assessed each year for worthiness to receive an award or move up the scale. In practice it is a matter of being in with the right people who will champion your claim. Lord Moran, who was (inevitably) the first chairman of the Advisory Committee on Distinction Awards, recalled, shortly before his death in 1977, how 'Each autumn I drove round the regions and looked up the local medical potentate. Each neighbourhood had someone of importance whose views could be trusted.' More recently the choice has been made in a slightly less nepotic and haphazard fashion.

Regional juntas made up of senior existing members of the merit club propose new candidates for C awards to the central committee. Teaching hospitals, and similar prestigious establishments, have direct access to the committee, and, moreover, are offered three or four times more 'places' per 100 aspirants within their patronage. The central committee dispenses A and B awards in its own wisdom, largely relying upon the old boy network for inspiration. Ellis Downes said, 'I know of one anaesthetist who sits on a merit award committee who does more private work than anybody else. All the surgeons ask him to do their private lists because they know that next time the committee considers who might be next in line their name might be mentioned, and if they keep in with old Bloggsy, they'll do very well. It's not corruption, because, on the face of it, there's nothing corrupt taking place. But when you start to look below the surface it begins to look very sinister.' I don't know how Dr Downes was so well-informed about the composition of a secretive committee, or on the volume of private work undertaken by one of its members. But whether his allegations were well-based or simply a product of unsubstantiated pub gossip doesn't matter. What does matter is that this exceptionally intelligent and street-wise young doctor should be ready to take such a cynical view of the way his preceptors conduct their affairs.

The result of this *duce*-dominated system is that a grossly disproportionate share of awards is collared by practitioners of the more revered specialties (like heart physicians and brain surgeons, and, now, transplanters) working in high-hat places. Thus London, Oxford and Cambridge do twice or thrice as well as Sheffield or Leeds, particularly when it comes to the major awards, and chest surgeons do over three times as well as psychiatrists, with geriatricians hardly figuring in the list. This bias can hardly be unrelated to the fact that the central committee and its satellites (whose members are nominated by 'Central's' chairman) consist largely of physicians, surgeons and gynaecologists, this bracket of the clinical elite outnumbering humbler but no less valuable representatives of the trade (such as pathologists, psychiatrists and radiologists) by fourteen or fifteen to one on the patronage panels.

It has been argued that this apparent inequity merely reflects an unequal distribution of talent within the trade. It can equally well be argued that the system perpetuates such inequality. Excellent geriatricians are certainly of more value to the community than excellent brain surgeons, because while few of us ever need to have our brains sliced open, we all hope to grow old. But energetic high-flyers are likely to go for the posts and activities offering the highest honours and rewards. Ignoring, for the moment, foolish idealists like James Malone-Lee or Wendy Savage, it would seem obvious that the merit award system encourages a distortion of the pattern of medical care to the great disadvantage of the majority of the citizens who have to foot the bill.

Terence English doesn't agree. He's a transparently honest and caring man who believes 'passionately' that all doctors in the NHS should be paid the same salary, and he doesn't believe in 'tenure for life', but sees nothing wrong in the idea of extra rewards 'for those who happen to have worked particularly hard', whether in research, or clinical endeavour, or teaching, or even management. He's in favour of merit awards. 'There are injustices, but it's much better than using that relatively small sum of money to give everybody a little bit more.' He easily rejects the proposition that young doctors are attracted to certain specialties, not because they want to do them, but because in doing them they might end up with twice the salary and twice the pension of practitioners in other fields. 'You can argue that there's an undue number of awards in some specialties like cardiology and certain types of surgery. That happens. But what doesn't happen is that people go into those specialties because they think they'll be rewarded better as result of a merit award. That's peanuts compared to what they can earn out of private practice.' (This says quite a lot about the amount of money maximum-part-time consultants can garner from their private work. If a doubling of their NHS income because of the possession of an A-plus award is 'peanuts' compared to what they can earn in their private time, then they must be doing pretty well.) It is possible that Sir Terence English, viewing matters from his elevated state, doesn't quite appreciate the influence the prospect of awards may have upon the lower echelons of his profession.

The awards are secret. Recipients are not supposed to reveal their good fortune. There is no acknowledged parallel for this kind of disbursement of public money to unnamed beneficiaries. The condition was laid down upon the specious argument that, if identified, award holders would attract customers at the expense of their unhonoured fellows. However, a survey carried out a few years ago found that while over *two*-thirds of award *holders* wanted secrecy maintained, less than *one*-third of the unfavoured thought it appropriate. A measure pretending to safeguard the interests of the weaker brethen is, in fact, designed to protect the privileged from the jealousy and resentment of their neglected mates. It is, of course, absurd to suppose that patients, wholly ignorant of the devious ways of the profession, would nose around seeking out the As and the Bs and the Cs and the non-starters, distributing their custom accordingly.

But perhaps the worst feature of the merit award scheme is its deadening effect upon the imagination and will for innovation which ought to be among the most desirable characteristics of the young (fortyish) clinicians newly elected to the consultants' club. If they are to have a reasonable hope of pleasing their superiors, so gaining a substantial pay rise, they must keep quiet about the legitimate grievances of the Junior Hospital Doctors' league, from which they have just escaped, and they must not be seen to disturb the rules and interests of the first division team they have just joined.

In a critical article published in the *British Medical Journal* in 1975 two senior psychiatrists concluded that the merit award system 'means that elderly men continue to elect their own successors in perpetuity, and the repetition of existing patterns, right or wrong, is an inevitable consequence'. Nothing much has changed since then, except that 'Bevan's Gold' is now facing much more open criticism from both within and without the trade. In 1988, for example, the Review Body on Doctors' and Dentists' Remuneration, which, since 1971, has been the body responsible for making annual recommendations on the pay of the two professions (which the Government may or may not but usually does accept), suggested that merit awards, instead of being held for life (because they affect pensions as well as salaries) should be renewable at, say, five-yearly intervals, depending upon continuing good performance. The Review Body also thought it desirable to involve management in the selection process, so that awards would be more likely to go to consultants giving the NHS good value for money, and not just to the most 'clubbable' members of the club. It now seems possible that both these changes will be implemented.

Meanwhile, as a student you still have to toady to your betters in order to stand half a chance of obtaining a first job in a blue-ribbon hospital, which is the first rung on the Moran ladder. Then, for the next ten or fifteen years, you must sustain the sycophancy as you now slowly climb towards the consultants' bar. And having eventually clambered over that (and while now fairly safe from falling off, except by reason of certified insanity, or conviction for murder, or some equally unignorable grave fault, like grossly upsetting your elder brethren) you must carry on soft-soaping, and wearing the right ties, and voicing 'sound' opinions if you hope to climb any higher, and certainly if you aim to reach the top.

The Star Chamber

Insofar as doctors can still claim to be members of a self-regulating profession (now that politicians – 'He who pays the piper' – are exercising more and more control over the pattern of their activities), the General Medical Council is the *fons et origo* of their corporate being.

This Star Chamber of the profession was established by Act of Parliament in 1858 (the first of the now confusingly many medical Acts). It is officially a committee of the Privy Council, although its members are not, except by rare chance, Privy Councillors. But such is the charm and confusion of our non-existent but well-established British constitution.

The new body was charged with the task of maintaining the newly created Medical Register, and, as a corollary, was made the legal guardian of medical education and medical discipline, having the power to define what kind of qualification should be required in those seeking a listing in the roll of approved practitioners, and the additional power of 'striking off' those registered who subsequently were shown to have clay feet.

Before the Medical Act of 1978 the GMC consisted of forty-seven sages of whom only eleven were elected by the medical *hoi polloi* by means of a postal ballot of the whole profession, the rest (including three lay members) being appointed by the Queen, by those universities having medical faculties, and by the Royal Colleges. Most of the appointed members were hospital-based luminaries of a kind who love committee work, and, indeed, any kind of opportunity for parading wisdom and exercising power, and who probably had an A or A-plus merit award safely tucked underneath the belt. Even the elected minority were of the same kidney, because Dr Pillmonger of Pinner would never have heard of Dr Softwords of Solihull, who might have decided to put himself forward as a candidate, and so those members of the medical electorate who did trouble to return their forms (about one in three) almost invariably put their crosses against the names of contenders sponsored by the BMA (the Ordinary Doctors' Org) for want of any better guidance. And the BMA, of course, always put forward its own committee men and women – doctor-politicians liable to be more interested in the resonance of their own voices than the welfare of the profession at large, let alone its customers.

It was a thoroughly self-satisfied, almost self-selected junta whose members exemplified an attitude lambently expressed by Lord Platt, President of the Royal College of Physicians from 1957 to 1962, and a worthy treader in the footsteps of Moran. In an almost unbelievably arrogant statement the noble healer said, 'It is important that the government of the profession should not be too democratic. It should be aware of the views of all its members, but should take its standards from the top and clearly favour that small and not usually vocal minority whose professional standards, be it in practice or research, stand far above the average.'

However, this haughty conclave was soon to encompass its own deflation and dilution, partly because of its ham-fisted and archaic handling of a series of infamous disciplinary proceedings, and partly because it started demanding money from the peasants it controlled.

Up until 1969 most registered medical practitioners rarely spared the GMC a thought. Most would have been hard put to it to name the president of the day. On qualification they had paid £5 to get registered – and that was that. Thereafter, unless taken in adultery with a patient, or otherwise found out, they had no further contact with the body. Hardly any of them imagined they would receive one of those awesome letters from the registrar saying a complaint had been laid and coldly inviting a response. The other two functions of the Council – maintaining a Register and controlling the medical curriculum – appeared not to touch their lives. Then the Council announced that it was deep in the red at the bank. It needed a lot of ready cash to clear the overdraft, and another lot of ready cash to finance its new-found interest in organizing postgraduate education and certification. Therefore the Council (which is financed entirely from various fees received) proposed to charge each doctor in the land a trifling £2 a year for having his name kept on the Register.

The profession shook with rage. Out of 12,000 doctors polled by the magazine *World Medicine* (now defunct), 11,500 said they would not pay. This was no mere stinginess, but resentment at a charge designed to bring the Council in an extra £130,000 a year (its *current* income tops the £5 million mark) which nobody believed would be profitably spent. Inevitably, the protesters caved in. It was easier to sign a £2 cheque and send it off without the knowledge of your peers rather than run the risk of finding yourself hauled up for posing as a registered practitioner when not entitled so to do. But, at a stroke, the Council had made itself the most unpopular body on the medical scene, and thereafter its every move was keenly and critically scrutinized by its reluctant underwriters.

A number of subversives managed to get themselves elected to the Council through the postal ballot of the profession at large, so that the august body found itself subjected to more and more open criticism from both within and without its ranks. Soon dissatisfaction with the Council's oligarchic ways had reached a pitch which could no longer be ignored, and the Government announced the setting-up of an Inquiry into the Regulation of the Medical Profession under the chairmanship of Dr (later Sir Alec) Merrison, then Vice-Chancellor of Bristol University, and a physicist, not a medical man.

Merrison recommended not just more elected members of the GMC, but an elected *majority*. A new Medical Act was passed in 1978 which took account of his findings, and the following year a new Council assembled, its membership enlarged from forty-six to ninety-three, of whom fifty had been chosen by the proles. The fifty included several doctors from overseas, so that the large corps of Commonwealth medical immigrants were represented for the first time.

Among other changes the Disciplinary Committee was renamed the Professional Conduct Committee, and the previous only charge at its disposal – that of 'infamous conduct in a professional sense' – was changed to one of 'serious professional misconduct'. These were purely cosmetic changes, designed to emphasize the Council's role in maintaining high standards of medical practice rather than merely harassing wretched sinners.

The beauty of the old and all-embracing charge was that it allowed the lords of the profession to chuck out any member of the trade they didn't like, for, as Lord Justice Lopes said in 1894, 'If a medical man in the pursuit of his profession had done something in regard to it which will be reasonably regarded as disgraceful or dishonourable by his professional brethren of good repute and competency, then it is open to the General Medical Council, if that be shown, to say that he has been guilty of infamous conduct in a professional respect.'

Changing the charge to one of 'serious professional misconduct' doesn't alter the fact that the moguls can decide from time to time (or from case to case, for that matter) what constitutes the crime.

Your ordinary courts have far less discretion and wield far less power. You are either found guilty of murder or you are not. You are either found guilty of illegal parking or you are not. In either case, before you can be penalized, it has to be shown that you have broken a well-defined and written law, and the maximum penalty has been by Parliament decreed, and that maximum is graded according to the perceived gravity of the offence. You can't be sent to prison for parking on a double yellow line. (Unless, of course, you refuse to pay the fine.)

Not so at the GMC. The Council regularly distributes a booklet to all doctors outlining its current thinking on professional misconduct and listing the commonest errors of behaviour likely to attract its condemnation. As recently as 1970 this *Best Sins Guide* reminded the peasantry that a doctor (in the last century) had had his name erased from the Register for keeping and exhibiting 'an anatomical museum containing waxworks of a disgusting character'. This might have been put in as a bit of a joke, designed to lighten the tone of a pretty threatening and dismal document, but I don't think so. The councillors and their staff are not a notably jokey lot (or certainly weren't twenty years ago). I think it was put in to make the point that the list of sins provided was by no means comprehensive, and that anybody could be had up for any kind of deviant behaviour – deviant, that is to say, from the kind of orthodoxy espoused by the top brass.

Not all the victims of the Council's wrath have been arraigned on such outrageous grounds, but in view of the fact that the overt purpose of the Council's being is the protection of the public against incompetents, charlatans and rogues, it is interesting to note how its well-nigh open-ended disciplinary powers have been exercised over the years.

In theory the Council does not initiate proceedings, and only acts upon complaints received, but it not infrequently gets round this annoying restriction by arranging for some other body (even, at times, its own solicitors) to lay the necessary information. It is also automatically notified whenever a doctor is convicted of a criminal offence. (Which is why, for example, a doctor's signature is accepted as a good supporting guarantee on a passport application form. It's not because doctors are regarded as sea-green incorruptibles, but because they stand to lose so much if caught out in a misdemeanour.)

Immense and almost autocratic power lies in the hands of the president, who, by himself, or by delegation, acts a procurator-fiscal, senior judge and foreman of the jury. He it is who first considers complaints received, and chooses whether or not to take any notice of them. If he decides to go ahead, the doctor gets a letter outlining the allegation and inviting comment. The charge and the doctor's response is then considered in private by a small Preliminary Proceedings Committee (PPC), which may or may not decide that the matter should then proceed to a full public hearing before the nineteen-strong Professional Conduct Committee (PCC, which the president may or may not choose to chair, depending on the importance of the case. (He did in the recent well-publicized matter of the 'Kidneys for Sale' affair.)

The Council receives over 1,000 complaints each year, most of which, in the words of its president, Sir Robert Kilpatrick, 'don't provide even a scrap of evidence which could stand up against the doctor, and no action is recommended'. In 1989 the PPC considered

123 cases, of which forty-two were referred to the PCC. Apart from such referrals, or a decision to take no action, the PCC may send the accused a letter of advice or admonition, or invoke the Council's health procedures (see below). So careful screening and investigation has already taken place before anybody faces public trial.

The PCC is like a court of law to the extent that the unfortunate prisoner in the dock is questioned before his accusers by an experienced advocate, witnesses may be subpoenaed, evidence is given on oath, and the accused may also be represented by a legal eagle.

The PCC is far removed from a court of law to the extent that the nineteen judges (who are also the jurors) have no legal training or experience, may be wholly unsuited to the task of weighing the evidence presented by a cunning lawyer, and, in determining guilt, are not required to be satisfied that the poor wretch before them has broken some written or established rule, for it is sufficient that they should disapprove of what has allegedly occurred. It is true that lay magistrates may also dispense justice with less than professional expertise, but they *are* bound by a pretty comprehensive and detailed set of precedents and precepts, and they cannot deprive someone of his livelihood simply because they don't much care for the cut of his jib, and their crasser decisions can readily be modified by a higher court.

It is true, also, that a condemned doctor can appeal against sentence to the Judicial Committee of the Privy Council, but, apart from correcting evident travesties of natural justice or the results of grossly negligent or unlawful proceedings, how can a bunch of elderly and eminent lawyers question judgments about what constitutes 'serious professional misconduct' arrived at by a bunch of eminent and elderly doctors? Appeals hardly ever succeed. (I have to admit that, these days, most of the members of the GMC are a good deal younger than I am, but that doesn't apply to the members of the Judicial Committee of the Privy Council. And in any case, it's not how old you are, but how old you think and act.)

So how has Lord Platt's 'small and not usually vocal minority whose professional standards stand far above the average' tended to define 'serious professional misconduct'?

Up until quite recently the moguls have been most disturbed by crimes such as adultery with patients (or some allied sport), or being drunk in charge (of a car or a customer), or advertising, or knocking a competitor. The largest emphasis has been placed on the kind of behaviour which could interfere with trade. Adultery with a patient interferes with trade because if people get the idea that their friendly neighbourhood physician may be a philanderer they will be less willing to let the doctor come and go unhindered, and to visit, say, the mistress of the house while the master is at the office. Advertising has always received the full treatment. When Charles Hill (later Lord Hill of Luton) made his voice famous during World War II as the 'Radio Doctor' he was not named, on the specious grounds that, if identified, he might attract customers from rivals in his parish. Rubbish, of course, because, apart from the fact that he was then employed full-time as secretary of the BMA, and not interested in attracting patients of any kind, nobody could mistake the voice, which was of a kind which once heard is never fogotten.

That's just one simple example of the absurdity of the rules then governing the profession. They were designed to protect the selfish interests and public image of its members (and, more particularly, its leading members) and were directed hardly at all (except by coincidence) towards the common weal.

Changes are taking place. Outsiders are demanding that the GMC should become more concerned with monitoring and jumping on professional incompetence instead of concentrating upon ungentlemanly behaviour. In 1989, for example, the deaf MP, Jack Ashley, suggested that doctors who over-prescribe tranquillizers, and automatically issue repeat prescriptions for these dangerous drugs, should be disciplined by the Council. This is to misunderstand that body's powers and functions, which, though large, are also strictly circumscribed.

Sir Robert Kilpatrick explains. 'By Act of Parliament we have a procedure with very strict procedural rules, and the charge of "serious professional misconduct" is the only charge we *can* bring. It's been enshrined in all the Acts since 1858. That doesn't mean there may not be a case for change, but we can't change at a whim. We have to change the Act, which means there has to be new legislation. That's often not realized by journalists and many members of the public. They know, for example, that in the courts a charge of manslaughter may be changed to one of dangerous driving, and don't understand that we don't have that option. We only have that one charge so far as conduct is concerned, and one other separate procedure which is that the individual is seriously impaired by reason of some physical or mental condition – our health procedures.'

The GMC's health procedures, established by the Act of 1978, do represent a considerable humanizing of the Council's policing functions. Doctors whose performance falls below safe and acceptable standards by reason of 'ill health' – almost always meaning 'mental illness', and almost always involving alcohol or other drug abuse – can be reported to the Council's Health Committee. But, instead of facing the normal penal investigations and proceedings, they can be urged to seek treatment and advice from nominated physicians within their region, or to continue under the care of a doctor they may already have consulted. So long as they follow the proposals of the Health Committee, which may include a restriction on the nature of their practice, or a requirement that they should only work under supervision, or even a suspension of their registration, no further formal steps are taken. Most doctors brought to the Committee's attention (and there were only thirty in 1989 who were invited to undergo medical examination) accept the guidance offered. A small rump, who have refused or been unable to cooperate in the first and voluntary stages of the 'health procedures', are required to appear before the Health Committee, whose proceedings are private and not reported in the press. The Committee may formally suspend a doctor's registration, or make it conditional, for periods limited by law (with a review required after those limits have expired). Only these facts are reported to prospective employers, and no details of the doctor's 'difficulties' are disclosed. To this extent, at least, the Council is attempting to differentiate between the 'mad' and the 'bad'.

But back to the main issue. Sir Robert acknowledges that 'there is a great deal of concern at the fact that we can only find that there has been serious professional misconduct, or there has not, and that we can't deal with a lesser charge. I think it's about a different charge, and we're now looking at that very actively.' He points out that a charge of serious professional conduct relates only to some specific incident in the doctor's career, which may give some indication of his general competence and behaviour, but which may equally well be an isolated lapse in a generally worthy record of performance. Erasure from the Register is not (in theory, at least) a 'punishment' for a professional sin, but a measure aimed at protecting the public from a person judged not fit to remain in practice. Moreover, it is a devastating sanction. 'A doctor whose name has been erased may supplicate to get back on the Register at a later stage,' comments Sir Robert, 'but if he has been erased for longer than a few months he virtually never gets back into employment as a medical practitioner, at least in terms of clinical care. And if he's under forty-five or fifty that's a very serious penalty. You stop a working lifetime.' The Council is therefore, and rightly, reluctant to find that a particular offence, even if proved 'beyond reasonable doubt', does indeed amount to 'serious professional misconduct' unless it is of such gravity or of such a nature that it does indicate that the miscreant is not fit to pursue his trade.

There can be no doubt that up until quite recently the Council has exercised its disciplinary powers more in defence of the profession's private interests and image, than to protect the public from incompetents (hence the case of the 'disgusting waxworks' and the emphasis upon such venial sins as advertising and knocking colleagues). But there is equally no doubt that a reformed and broader-based body has become more aware of its proper function as an agent of the common weal, and its critics perhaps fail to give it sufficient credit for attempting to function in a more enlightened fashion under archaic rules of procedure.

The Council has been accused of resisting change. Sir Robert denies this, pointing out that it wouldn't be very sensible for a statutory body to make a change of policy 'on a whim', and without a great deal of consideration, later finding that it had 'to eat its words'. It is working on, and, he believes, will soon have evolved, a satisfactory scheme (which would have to *appear* satisfactory to, *inter alia*, the politicians, who will have to enshrine its proposals in the law) for monitoring and dealing with doctors whose performance is 'professionally unacceptable', rather than having to wait until sub-standard practitioners do some one thing so clearly and appallingly blameworthy that they can be brought under control by a charge of 'serious professional misconduct'.

Sir Robert favours a mechanism which would be analogous to the present health procedures, whereby informal informations and enquiries and persuasions could be expected to help, and protect from further trouble and deterioration, a majority of incompetents, leaving only a hard core to face compulsory supervision, or further training, or suspension, or whatever.

If this can be achieved, then the GMC will become better placed than ever before to fulfil its chief and proper purpose. But it will cost a lot of money, and the annual registration fee will have to be hyped by a good deal more than the inflation rate. Let's hope that doesn't cause another peasants' revolt. Perhaps it's time the taxpayer made a contribution. After all, the Council is supposed to exist for the taxpayers' benefit, and not for that of the medical trade. Its self-financing status hasn't noticeably insulated the profession from the influence of the State.

Other Constraints

The GMC may be the principal agency for controlling the behaviour of the medical profession, and the most overtly powerful because of its ability to chuck people out of the trade, but it is by no means the only constraining influence upon the doctors' preciously regarded but largely illusory right to 'clinical freedom', by which is meant that every practitioner is entitled, and solely within his own judgment, to decide how best to deal with each of his customers, without let or hindrance from any other person or body corporate. Such a concept, for many a practical and social reason, has never been more than a happy myth, but the nature of the constraints on 'clinical freedom' have changed from time to time.

British doctors in the pre-NHS era, for example, couldn't prescribe treatments which their customers couldn't possibly afford. (Well, they could have done, but it wouldn't have been much use.) In effect the initiation of the service, which was at first regarded by the profession as a threat to its autonomy, gave doctors far more 'clinical freedom' than they had ever experienced before. At last they could do their best for their customers without regard to the overwhelming damper of immediate costs. And that is why, with forty-years'-plus experience of the system, a rather myopic and slow-thinking profession has been converted from a shrill opponency to an equally shrill championship of the ship in which it serves.

But the open-ended commitment of the Government, as provided by law, to serve the medical needs of citizens, as and how they might arise, has become increasingly costly and difficult to preserve, and as the original fallacy that the NHS would shortly 'pay for itself' by making everybody healthier, and thus reducing demand, has been shown to be untrue, the moneymasters have found it more and more necessary to exercise control.

They haven't yet quite discovered how to do this, but there is an increasing recognition, both within and without the medical profession, that the costs and activities of the nation's largest industry do have to be 'managed' and made 'cost-effective'. Doctors can no longer expect to be allowed just to do their own thing. They have to show that they are giving value for money received and spent.

Family Health Services Authorities exercise some kind of control over the quality of general practice. They can inspect premises and, after due warning, abort contracts with practitioners who don't come up to standard in terms of the facilities and services they provide. But FHSAs are often hampered by necessity. They are required to organize the provision of general medical services within their bailiwick, and will sometimes, for example, tolerate the services of not markedly excellent practitioners from overseas, operating, perhaps, from poor premises, simply because they are speaking the language and understanding the special problems of their immigrant constituents. And who's to say that's wrong? Doctors are for people, after all.

Just like the GMC, FHSAs have been accused of failing to bring to book doctors who clearly, upon the evidence, have given their customers a raw deal. Again, such complaints are often the result of a perfectly understandable misunderstanding of the role and powers of the authority concerned.

Anybody feeling aggrieved by the treatment (medical or personal) they've experienced at the hands of their friendly neighbourhood GP can lodge a complaint with the local FHSA, hoping for an acknowledgment of fault and an apology. They often don't get either, and this is because the committee which considers the complaint is not interested in deciding whether or not the doctor concerned has done a bad thing, but simply and purely whether or not he has broken his contract with the FHSA.

The commonest complaint received by FHSAs is that a doctor has failed to answer a request for a home visit upon the occasion of a real or feared 'emergency'. If that be proved, then he may be fined, and if his apparent dereliction of duty has been so gross that the fine exceeds a certain sum, the fact is reported to the Health Department which, in turn, passes the information to the GMC.

But supposing a doctor does in fact turn up on a home visit, possibly half-sloshed, and is abusive to all concerned for calling him out, and then diagnoses indigestion in a patient with chest pain, who dies from a coronary thrombosis (which was the true cause of the chest pain) half an hour after the doctor has left, and whose life might have been saved by a good diagnosis and prompt action, then there may be no sustainable cause for complaint.

The doctor (and I hope there now are now very few of his sort – well, there's no harm in hoping) has fulfilled the terms of his contract by 'turning out', and the fact that he did a thoroughly rotten job of work is not a matter which the old Family Practitioner Committees have been inclined to contemplate. This may be changing. Barry Salter finds that both the lay and medical members of investigating committees are more ready to question a GP's clinical judgment than they were five or ten years ago. But to attract admonition (let alone a fine for breach of contract), the culprit would have to have displayed a degree of incompetence or carelessness clearly inconsistent with accepted standards of practice. It is not enough simply to show that he's made a mistake. If the attitude of FHSAs towards professional competence is indeed becoming more rigorous, that would reflect the growing general awareness (both within and without the profession) of the need for a constant evaluation of standards and performance. No doctor is an island, entire of it self. Not any more.

(FHSAs are not just FPCs with a new name. They also have a new structure. There are fewer members and those remaining are now to be paid a handsome retainer of £5,000 a year, with chair-persons earning £10,000, which suggests that the Government intends that these bodies should be required to work quite hard for their living and be seen to exercise control.)

Rudeness to patients is not a breach of contract, though many may feel it ought to be, but Barry Salter points out that an abrasive attitude could prevent a doctor from rendering his customers an adequate service, and notorious offenders may have their attention drawn to this possible consequence.

Hospital doctors, including consultants, come under the control of health service managers and the appropriate health authority. When the NHS began, the medical pattern of hospital life was largely determined by the consultants. Matron ruled supreme over the nurses, brooking small interference from 'outsiders', including the medical staff. A civilian House Governor or Hospital Secretary looked after the fabric and general administration.

In 1974 so-called consensus management was born, with an administrator, a treasurer, a medical officer and a nursing officer sitting together and striving to agree on how things should be done in their health district. A thumbs-down response from any one of the four could block the contrivings of the rest.

In 1983, in an increasingly desperate effort to improve 'efficiency' (which really means to contain costs), general managers were appointed to take day-to-day decisions at the various levels of administration. A good many of this new breed of hospital animal were administrators promoted from the old consensus teams. Some doctors, treasurers and even a few nurses were appointed to these posts, but quite a few incumbents were imported from outside the NHS – ex-Army officers and businessmen – with the idea that such captains of men and industry would give the complacent natives the kind of shake-up they so richly deserved. This produced consider-able resentment. The immigrant bosses often had small understand-ing of the nature and needs of the professionals they were expected to control, which meant that they couldn't command the essential cooperation of the troops, and many soon left.

James Malone-Lee, admitting the need for strong leadership of a quality able to counteract the paralysing bickerings and jockeyings for advantage indulged in by the many vested interests which make up the hospital world, says, 'I knew the Army people wouldn't last long. People are now beginning to understand that if you're going to have effective management, it will have to come from within the NHS. There's a feeling that people in the NHS can't be much good, because if they were they wouldn't be there on that kind of salary, but somewhere else, with a company car and so on. That's a most contemptible myth. People fail to realize that there are highly talented managers in the Health Service who could earn very respectable salaries elsewhere, but choose not to because they're motivated by other principles . . . We've had a terribly rough decade, but out of the ashes are coming some very tough, determined and committed people who've taken a hell of a bashing, but are still there, and they're going to do the Health Service an immense amount of good because of their quality. It's been very interesting to see all the damp kippers from industry scuttling back to run buses or whatever, while the tougher individuals stay behind. So I don't feel so despondent about it all.'

These progressive changes in administrative structure have led to a parallel erosion of the consultant's erstwhile status as supreme ruler of his own small kingdom or 'firm'. He has had to modify his activities more and more in response to managerial decisions concerning the use and scale of resources, and to undertake a deputed managerial responsibility himself so that his department is run according to guidelines set from above, and, perhaps most importantly, to accept the use of various devices aimed at monitoring performance and the value and effectiveness of the work of his team.

The consultant's erstwhile autarchy has been further modified by schemes designed to encourage the best use of what's available, and to avoid wasteful overlapping of functions and effort. Thus a number of hospitals have recently appointed 'clinical directors' to oversee and coordinate the activities of departments, such as cardiology or paediatrics, or whatever, which employ a number of consultants and their acolytes. The directors are not chosen on grounds of seniority, but because they are the sort of people most likely to be acceptable to their colleagues, and therefore most likely to succeed in the difficult task of getting them to work together instead of in a spirit of unprofitable competition.

Apart from increasing managerial and clinical control, consultants are by no means immune from disciplinary procedures (and quite apart from professional crimes of a kind which might bring them under the heavy hand of the GMC). The Regional Health Authorities can, and do, suspend consultants from their jobs while complaints about their competence and behaviour are 'investigated', and the tortuous procedure which then follows can keep a good doctor in limbo for years (albeit on full pay) and finally destroy a hard-won career.

Consultants, by the very nature of the competition they have had to survive in order to achieve their posts, are unlikely to be incompetents. They may, like the rest of us, occasionally go mad or take to the bottle, but, such risks apart, there is small chance that a consultant becomes unable to deliver good, informed medical care, although an individual may become indifferent to or lazy in the task.

What can quite easily happen is that a consultant can anger and irritate the medical establishment by expressing unorthodox views or otherwise rocking the boat. Most suspensions of consultants have occurred because of complaints from their colleagues, rather than patients or management, or because issues like the Cleveland child abuse affair have frightened the employing authorities into action.

Wendy Savage was suspended because her seniors at the London Hospital disapproved of her liberal attitudes towards the handling of pregnancy and childbirth (attitudes which will almost certainly become the orthodoxy within the next ten years). Her views simply conflicted too strongly with those of the bosses, who decided to try to rid themselves of an irritant. Marietta Higgs was barred from her main occupation because she had become a popular hate figure, and not because of any suggestion of professional incompetence or lack of diligence and integrity. Whether or not all her diagnoses of possible sexual abuse in her young patients were correct, nobody, today, would be outraged by the kind of vigorous investigation of an evil phenomenon which led to her conflict with authority. We've got used to the sad idea that she may have been more or less right. Both women, being exceptionally strong characters, have survived their ordeals, emerging with heads bloodied but unbowed. A disturbing number of less tough-minded specialists have been destroyed by similarly ill-judged attacks.

Short of formal proceedings, Regional Medical Officers, who are full-time bureaucrats, may 'carpet' consultants who step out of line.

For example, a distinguished Cambridge cardiologist who has campaigned, on legitimate scientific grounds, against the 'harvesting' of organs for transplantation from living but so-called 'brain-dead' donors, was told by his RMO to keep his unwelcome views to himself, and to refrain from talking to the press. He complied, at least to the extent of making his campaigning more discreet, and later took early retirement. Had he not observed the warning then, presumably he too might have faced suspension – simply for voicing a respectable and honestly held opinion.

But disciplinary procedures, whether instituted by the GMC, or by FHSAs, or by Regional Health Authorities, are the least important of the factors influencing medical behaviour. Much more cogent is the new concept that doctors and departments and institutions have a duty to monitor their own performance, or allow other kinds of experts, such as economists, to do it for them, and then to modify their activities in the light of what's been found. It's a blindingly simple and obviously sound approach to improving standards and results, but one which has only now gained general acceptance, and now only because the costs of medical care are so high and rising all the time that the people who dispense the cash (the Government here, and the insurers in the USA) are being forced to discover how to use every penny to the best advantage. There is also the fact that modern technology has only recently made it possible to assemble and analyse the vast quantities of information needed to produce an accurate picture of what is going on.

'Medical audit' is the buzz phrase of the decade. At the simplest level a GP or specialist will look at his results and costs (in terms of time and effort as well as money) and compare them to those of his peers, and, if they are better or worse, endeavour to find out why.

A Newcastle hospital is checking up on ex-patients six months and two years after discharge in an attempt to discover how they're functioning in society. A few years ago any hospital would have been content to judge its performance by the proportion of clients it could send home on their own two feet, and wouldn't have thought it necessary to establish whether its procedures were truly useful and cost-efficient in terms of restoring patients to a normal or worthwhile life.

Sociologists and economists have increasingly taken an interest in health affairs, and, in an attempt to quantify the value of various medical procedures, have invented a number of indices, amongst the best-known of which are QALYs.

A QALY is a 'quality-adjusted life year', and is designed to take into account not just survival, but the survivor's degree of well-being. A year of perfect health would score 1, whereas a year of 50 per cent disability would score 0.5. A procedure can then be assessed in terms of the cost of each QALY it produces (the cost of the procedure divided by the QALY count). Thus a recently published table, listing about a dozen common medical interventions, estimated that each QALY gained by a hip replacement costs £750, whereas each heart transplant QALY costs £5,000. A kidney transplant QALY comes out at £3,000, but the same patient treated in hospital on a kidney machine once or twice a week would cost £14,000 per QALY gained. The cheapest QALYs of all are the fruit of preventive medicine. Nobody is suggesting that hip replacements should be abandoned, and the money saved be ploughed into anti-smoking clinics, for other considerations, such as the need to relieve present suffering, are clearly just as important as getting the best value for money in terms of the overall improvement of the national health. But the approach does help an informed assessment of what we are getting for the money spent, and, further researched and refined, QALYs and other methods for costing and evaluating procedures will undoubtedly be used to help determine how doctors may be best employed.

The critical judgment of performance and the requirement that standards must be met are now central features of the medical life. Clinical freedom, if it ever existed, is a phrase which is rapidly acquiring a pretty hollow ring.

6   *Educating Doctors*

Perhaps the most serious criticism of the proudly 'self-regulating' medical profession, is that it has failed to train its neophytes in a manner appropriate to the functions they are going to be called upon to fulfil. But that's what happens when you give experts in one field of endeavour (such as diagnosing and treating heart disease) dominance over another (like education), which they don't understand and sometimes may not even care about very much.

If a first-class honours geography graduate decides that he'd like to teach his subject to ten-year-olds, he goes away for a year and gets himself a postgraduate certificate in education. If an experienced ward sister wants to become a sister-tutor she has to take a similar intensive course in the tricks of the teaching trade. Yet it is assumed that a physiologist or a neurologist or a biochemist or a heart surgeon (and just because he knows his subject very well) can stroll into the lecture room and make a proper job of passing on wisdom and learning. This is rubbish. There *are* a few natural-born teachers who can be effective without any special training, but even the most talented amongst them could do better still if versed in modern educational theory and techniques.

Terence English recalls a 'teach-in' with medical students in Cambridge. 'We had to cover the whole field of congenital heart disease between 2.30 and 5 in one afternoon, and that was the only exposure they were going to get on the subject. So we got together a radiologist and a cardiologist and a pathologist and myself. I think we provided a tremendous programme, but they obviously came out of it completely bog-eyed because of the sheer amount of information involved.'

So here were four good men and true, putting a lot of effort into what we may be sure was a competent and possibly brilliant exposition of a complex topic, but accomplishing far less than they had hoped because they were attempting too much. A trained teacher or educationalist knows, more or less, how much learning your average pupil can be expected to acquire in the course of an afternoon, or a week, or a year, or an entire school and university career. He also recognizes the crucial difference between learning and knowledge.

In the old days the only way to acquire a medical 'education' was to attach yourself to a practising physician, and to follow him around, observing his methods and attitudes, then going off and doing likewise (with, perhaps, a few personal variations).

This medieval pattern of craft apprenticeship was still extant when the GMC was created in 1858 and given the task of determining what kind of training should fit a person to be included on its register. But professions (or, at least, those members of a guild who are already well-established in the club) like to make entry as difficult and onerous as may be, if only to increase their own honour and advantage, and so it became a requirement that supplicants for entry to the medical trade should demonstrate great learning before being admitted as fellows.

The trouble was that, in 1858, there wasn't a great deal of learning to be had. Nobody knew anything about vitamins or hormones or DNA, or even quite how women became pregnant (they knew how to *make* it happen, all right, but had small idea of what actually goes on). What they did know about was anatomy, because countless eager researchers over the ages had cut up corpses, and looked at fragments of flesh through one of those new-fangled microscopes, and described and named the bits and pieces they had found in minute detail, commonly giving them thoroughly unhelpful esoteric dog Latin or eponymous labels (such as 'extensor carpi radialis brevis' for a small muscle in the hand, and 'the crypts of Lieberkühn' for minute, tube-like depressions in the lining of the intestines first described in the eighteenth century by the said Herr Professor Lieberkühn), but often without much, if any, understanding of what the various components of the body beautiful were for, let alone how they worked.

Such Latinization of the catalogue of body parts may have served a useful purpose when that tongue was the only *lingua franca* of the educated classes, so that anatomists and doctors and students in Moscow, Paris and London could equally identify a small muscle identified as 'extensor carpi radialis brevis', but those days have long since disappeared. I (reluctantly and inefficiently) learnt Latin at school because, when I was a boy, it was supposed to be a *sine qua non* of a young gentleman's education, and you couldn't opt out, at least until you'd reached the fifth form. So when I got to medical school I at least knew that 'brevis' meant 'short' and could make some little sense out of labels like 'extensor carpi radialis brevis', and the same went for my contemporaries, all of whom would have endured a traditional public or, at the very least, grammar school education. Nowadays many bright students tackling the medical curriculum will never have handled a Latin grammar or painstakingly attempted to understand the jokes of Juvenal written in his native tongue, so they have to remember a long list of body parts described in terms which give them little clue to their place or function. This is one example of the manner in which an addiction to tradition seriously hampers learning. A new anatomical vocabulary is long overdue, but it is unlikely to emerge, because the immense labour involved wouldn't earn its inventor much credit. Finding out something new is mistakenly seen as far more valuable than the intelligent representation, organization and analysis of the knowledge we already have. We are awash with knowledge. We don't know how to handle it all.

Anyway, the anatomists' detailed descriptions constituted much of medical knowledge as it stood in 1858, and medical students were required (and in some schools still are) to be able, for example, to name and recognize any of the many small bones in the foot when a desiccated, isolated specimen of one of them is produced – despite the fact that such expertise could hardly help them serve their future customers. So, *faute de mieux*, anatomy became a dominant subject in the medical curriculum, and has remained so, with a disproportionate slice of the pre-clinical course still devoted to the laborious dissection of dried-out pickled corpses whose bits and pieces bear only a passing resemblance to the once-living flesh.

Certainly an orthopaedic surgeon should have an intimate grasp of the origins and insertions and relationships and courses and branches of the muscles, ligaments, nerves and vessels surrounding the knee joint, but to a family doctor or a psychiatrist or a brain surgeon the knowledge is quite useless, and the time to acquire such specialized learning is when a career as a sawbones has been chosen.

At any rate, the GMC of 1858, and successive Councils for the next 100 years, laid down, in their imagined wisdom, detailed and inflexible rules concerning the courses to be followed – so many hours to be spent on dissecting paupers' bodies, so many lectures on compounding salves and rolling pills, so much time to be spent at the lunatic asylum and the fever hospital and in the labour ward. It was all carefully calculated so that (in theory, anyway) no gaps remained in the web of understanding owned by the graduating doctor. The trouble is that (unlike law or theology) medicine has increased its skills and understandings at an exponential rate, so that the original aim of turning out a complete doctor at the time of graduation, who not only knew all the tricks of the trade, but also understood the whole of the known science lying behind the art, long ago became impossible. Yet the old-fashioned target stayed in place, with the result that the required pattern of study rapidly became absurdly overloaded, not only because the existing disciplines (like physiology and pharmacology) were expanding their knowledge-base almost by the hour, but also because newly important subjects (like biochemistry and bacteriology and radiology) were demanding their place in the undergraduate curriculum.

So the GMC ponderously strove to continue its detailed control over the way medical students should be taught long after the complexities of the task were beyond the understanding of most of its members. (I vividly remember one report on medical education compiled in the 1950s by eminent members of the guild – predominantly clinicians – which desperately strove to justify the requirement that entrants to the trade should have achieved an A-level – or, as it was then, Higher School Certificate – pass in physics on the sole grounds that doctors ought to understand how x-ray machines work and also the optics of lighting in operating theatres. The poor and expert darlings were clearly grasping at straws because they hadn't a clue about the nature and purpose of education.)

Nevertheless, these amateurs (or ignoramuses) exercised supreme control, and any school departing from the course prescribed ran the risk of finding its degree or diploma made worthless, and so, of course, none did depart, and there was no room for experiment or innovation.

Over the past quarter of a century this stranglehold has been progressively relaxed, so that the GMC's requirements are now couched in only the vaguest of terms, but the universities are only slowly recovering from the long tradition of stultifying conformity for which the GMC was totally responsible.

Not surprisingly, it is only the newer universities, with new medical faculties, such as Southampton, Nottingham and Leicester, which have taken much advantage of this new-found freedom. They have had the opportunity to plan their courses from scratch, and thus the ability to prune archaic elements of the traditional curriculum and to introduce new ones, without encountering resistance from entrenched interests. It is comparatively easy to tell the newly appointed professor of a new department of anatomy or surgery how much of the students' time and the school's budget he can command, and how many lecturers he can have. It is much more difficult to persuade an existing potentate to accept a diminution in his role in order to give new subjects space. So a student at, say, Leicester, is now getting a much better education than his contemporaries at some older and more celebrated and more hidebound institutions.

Bill Grove, as an undergraduate at the Royal Free in London, has small respect for the training he has received. As a pre-clinical student he was required to absorb and regurgitate masses of information which (or so it seemed to him) had little relevance to his future career. 'The biochemists tried to turn us into biochemists.' There were nods towards relevance. Sheets were distributed, outlining the aspects of the subject to be learned, and the bits most likely to be useful to a working doctor were starred. 'But we weren't told why, and were still required to know the pieces in between.'

His experience in the clinical years was not much better, not because his tutors tried to force too much information down his throat, but because they didn't try much at all. 'Registrars have so many commitments in terms of their duty to the NHS, and have to produce so much research in order to get on, with 60 per cent of people getting surgical consultancies now having PhDs', that it's not surprising that their teaching function comes low on the list of priorities.

'We spend half our time standing in wards waiting for people to turn up to teach us, and they don't turn up, and because you're medical students they don't even apologize to you. But if *you* don't turn up a ton of bricks comes down. I was on an obstetrician's firm for six weeks, and for five weeks he didn't turn up for his ward round, so on the sixth week I didn't turn up, and it was a great mistake.'

Royal Free students have an examination at the end of every term. 'Which means that a lot of what we're doing is rote-learning from textbooks so that we can regurgitate it at the exam. This takes the emphasis away from clinical skills. The University of London has warned medical schools in the last few years that clinical skills are not coming up to standard, and that the people failing finals are failing on clinical skills and not on knowledge. After four years of medicine I certainly don't feel confident about the straightforward examination of patients, which can't be right.'

Bill Grove complained of a lack of experience of many common but important illnesses because the beds of London teaching hospitals are largely occupied by patients suffering from 'very, very odd diseases. So you sit there with the registrar who says, "Now, imagine somebody comes in with X – what are you going to do?" You're having to *imagine* something you ought to be doing in practice. I know several people in their fifth year who've done ten to twelve weeks' surgery but who've never seen somebody with appendicitis.'

He sums it all up in lambent fashion. 'The course seems to be there as a sort of obstacle to becoming a doctor. There's a series of posts you have to get past, and fences you have to jump over, and then you're a doctor. But it doesn't actually seem to be a vehicle for turning somebody who isn't a doctor into somebody who is.'

These are not just the grumblings of rebellious youth. Dr Malone-Lee, with his experience in another prestigious London school, pretty well echoes Bill Grove's words and feelings. He believes that A-level students have 'an extraordinarily analytical approach to their learning . . . but we take these young people and then destroy this outlook by force-feeding them this vast amount of knowledge –

more than a person can possibly handle if they're to learn it by comprehension, so we force them into rote-learning. We expose students to increasingly large quantities of theoretical knowledge, so that more and more teaching takes place in the tutorial room rather than round the bed, and less and less emphasis is put on the clinical skills and communication skills that are required. . . . This is reflected in our examination results. We have quite a high failure rate of around 30 per cent, and they're coming down in clinical skills.'

Ellis Downes of Leicester has a different tale to tell. 'My first two years were very nice. You don't just do anatomy, physiology and biochemistry. In one term you might have the reproductive system. So you might have the anatomy of the female reproductive tract from 10 to 11, and the endocrinology from 11 to 12, and after lunch the physiology of reproduction – all very enjoyable.' But he still thinks he may have had to learn more than enough anatomy.

At Leicester students are encouraged, right from the start, to regard patients as people, rather than as vehicles of disease. A 'Man in Society' course occupies a remarkable 20 per cent of teaching time during the first two years, dealing with subjects like psychology, sociology, epidemiology, statistics, and the way medicine is practised in other countries. And, apart from the now fairly general brief attachment to a general practice, students are allocated to a patient in the community, whom they visit from time to time. 'So we found out that a patient wasn't just a body in a nice, clean hospital bed, but was Mrs Bloggs, actually crippled with arthritis and finding it hard to make a cup of tea.' Good clinical teaching, with only two students attached to a 'firm' (compared to the six common elsewhere), an elective period spent abroad (Ellis went to a remote bush hospital in Zambia), the availability of teaching aids like computers with which to play instructive 'games', a good deal of attention paid to 'hands-on' procedures, and other imaginative devices, combined to give this young doctor an enjoyable undergraduate life, approaching something much more like an education than the kind of half-hearted and poorly organized 'vocational training' offered by the common run of medical schools. But even he, knowing what he knows now, wonders whether he'd go into it again.

'My vision of what being a doctor would be like, and what it's actually like, are completely different. I had no idea. Neither did any of my contemporaries. . . . But the sad fact is that there are 4 million unemployed, and once you've been trained as a doctor you're never out of work, and even if you don't enjoy the job, it pays reasonably well.'

Bill Grove is asked to go back to his old school to talk to sixth-formers who want to do medicine. 'And now I always say I won't because I'd only put people off. So it's an odd position, because although I'm enjoying what I'm doing now, and look forward to a career in surgery, I wouldn't wish the course on any school-leaver.'

These reactions may, in part, simply reflect the common truth that most of us wouldn't have the courage to embark upon any major undertaking (such as getting married) if we fully appreciated in advance all the stresses and strains involved, but they must also say something about the crushing effect upon the spirit and the mind of the present medical curriculum, even in enlightened places such as Leicester. A paper published in the *British Medical Journal* in 1989 reported the drinking habits of 260 medical students. At least 34 per cent of the men and, more surprisingly, 43 per cent of the women exceeded the suggested safe weekly limits for alcohol intake, which is twenty-one measures of gin (or the equivalent) for males, and fourteen for females. More than half the group said that their drinking had affected their academic performance at some time, and seventeen said this happened frequently. The incidence of excessive drinking among the students was over double that found in the general population. If this bibulous life-style had been discovered largely in the men it might be considered a tribal phenomenon, with the lads merely striving to live up to the traditional if old-fashioned image of the macho, devil-may-care, rugger-playing, beer-swilling medical student. But the fact that the women outdid their male companions in the drinking stakes strongly suggests that the findings are symptomatic of distress caused by an inexcusably onerous and frustrating imposed regime.

Wendy Savage, now an elected member of the GMC, believes that it is not enough for the Council to be satisfied with giving medical schools a certain amount of flexibility. 'Instead of saying, "We've given them the opportunity and they haven't taken it", they should use their teeth and say, "You're not doing a good job here". We should be teaching students how to evaluate data critically – how to relate to people, because that's what they've got to do as doctors, and where to find the detailed information when they want it.' She has never forgotten one of her teachers, Donald Hunter, the father of industrial medicine, who said, 'You don't have to remember all these facts. All you have to know is where to look them up. What I want you to learn is how to think and analyse the data.'

I suspect that, since I spoke to her, Mrs Savage may have become more contented with the Council's attitude toward medical education, because her views are certainly shared by its present president. Sir Robert Kilpatrick is the Dean of Leicester University medical faculty, and was, in large part, responsible for designing the course which Ellis Downes has found has served him pretty well. And, before becoming president of the GMC, Sir Robert was chairman of its education committee. So his ideas tend to count.

'The striking difference between medical students and students doing physiology or genetics (or history, for that matter), is that the others don't attempt a complete coverage of their subject. They concentrate on the skeleton, with a fair amount of time spent on finding out about a particular part of it, and, in so doing, they find out how to find out and how to assess.

'Medical students don't get that. I see it every day. They don't know how our knowledge has been produced. . . . That's why medically qualified people so often say things you wouldn't expect members of the *public* to say. "Salt is bad for you" – doctors who say that cannot have even glanced at the evidence, which is that salt is bad for under 5 per cent of the population. They proceed to believe that salt is bad for 100 per cent – and this is a substance which is essential for health.'

The GMC issues recommendations on basic medical education every ten years, and the latest version was being prepared at the time I interviewed Sir Robert. He recalls how, as chairman of the education committee, he and his predecessor had received innumerable letters from individuals and organizations saying how important it was that students should know about legal medicine, or genito-urinary medicine, or AIDS, or social factors in disease, or whatever, and that the writer's pet subject could be covered in the course of a few lectures, so that it wasn't asking a lot to have it included in the list of required or recommended topics. 'The assumption is that the curriculum is like a passport, and that you just put stamps in saying "Done legal medicine", and so on [Bill Grove's 'posts' and 'fences']. That's a myth. That kind of teaching has no permanent effect at all. The psychological factors concerning memory are well known.'

Sir Robert expected the new recommendations to be based on the assumption that in future all doctors will undergo a minimum of four years' postgraduate training before being let loose on the public as fully independent operators. Much of their clinical and technical expertise would be acquired during this period, and the old and long-since unrealistic idea that the five undergraduate years must provide the student with all the skills and understandings needed for a lifetime's work would be buried for ever. Instead there would be a core curriculum (which all schools would be expected to adopt) and a series of options, so that a chosen field or fields of interest could be studied in depth and throughout the course, just as happens in other faculties. Undergraduates would no longer be required to have 'had a go' at a host of specialties, like radiology, or ear, nose and throat, or eyes, and so on, but could pick and choose 'the flavours that interested them', perhaps carrying on a particular study into the postgraduate years. As a result the student would end up with an education and a 'permanent legacy of enquiry', instead of becoming a confused and exhausted repository of largely forgotten and never fully comprehended information.

I found considerable sympathy among my respondents for the suggestion that medical students might benefit if their pre-clinical training was of a broader and less job-oriented nature, and was shared with students in other disciplines. According to Sir Robert several places are already very interested in the possibility, and at least one medical school has suggested a course in which the first two years are common to medicine, dentistry and biological science, with students having the opportunity to delay a final choice of career until the end of the introductory period. Ellis Downes wasn't too sure that medical students could happily share their instruction with students having different attitudes and interests, but was adamant in the view that the isolated, non-residential, London medical colleges are a disaster, and that all pre-clinical courses should be conducted in 'proper' universities, so that the neophyte doctor lives and eats and drinks and plays with a rich mix of his generation.

Why Be a Doctor?

Why do young people want to become doctors? And how are the few chosen from among the many who apply for places in medical schools?

When would-be medical students are interviewed they are inevitably asked why they fancy the profession, and a high proportion reply by claiming that they 'want to do good' and are inspired by the wish to 'help people'. Ra Gillon, as we have heard, believes this to be a genuine and entirely proper reason for the choice, but, as he points out, it is an answer which many latter-day interviewers (who are commonly high-powered academics wedded to the idea of medicine as a rigorous practical science rather than an art or a vocation) regard with some scepticism, believing it to be mouthed by aspirants who think that some such expression of high-minded intent is expected of them, or who can't think of a 'better' response, and who, it is assumed, haven't given the question the consideration it deserves. A minority of candidates (who may have been warned against the danger of appearing to be woolly-headed idealists) will have prepared a more down-to-earth and intellectually 'respectable' answer, claiming, perhaps, a desire to exploit an enthusiasm for the natural sciences, or saying they're excited by the potential of modern surgical techniques, or whatever. Such young sophisticates may score better with their hard-boiled inquisitors, but are not necessarily more soundly motivated than their apparently artless rivals.

I asked Bill Grove why *he* chose medicine. 'That's quite difficult to say. I was interested in sciences at school, but wasn't very good at maths, and medicine seemed to be a subject in which I could continue that interest without needing the kind of mathematical skills a pure scientist requires. Also medicine was a challenge. I didn't perform terribly well at school to begin with, although I gradually improved, and our careers advice teacher quoted medicine as a specific example of something not to aim for if you weren't capable of getting there, so I thought, "Well – I'll show them!" It really all happened by accident.'

Not much evidence of an early idealism or single-minded devotion to the idea of doctoring there, but Bill Grove went on to say that, having got into the medical game, he couldn't think of anything else he would want to do, and was now very keen to become a surgeon. He also said (surprisingly, in view of his criticism of the curriculum) that he 'couldn't imagine enjoying anything else as much as I've enjoyed the training I've done so far'.

Ellis Downes decided to be a doctor 'because my grandfather was a surgeon'. (Family medical connections are a frequently quoted determinant, although they may put young people off the trade as often as they turn them on.) 'But that wasn't really the reason why I went into medicine, although it did make me think along those lines. I knew I was always going to do something scientific, and I really like people and was attracted to a profession where you meet them every day. And there's a certain amount of romance involved. We all have this idea of a Dr Kildare-type figure, with nurses fluttering in the wings.'

So here are two young people who chose medicine with only the vaguest appreciation of what they were letting themselves in for, and who, in the light of experience, doubt whether they'd make the choice again, yet who wouldn't now opt out. Not all their contemporaries have proved so resilient, or concluded that the rewards of the medical life more than compensate for the tribulations, and the services of an organization which advises recently qualified doctors on how to switch to quite different alternative careers are said to be in brisk demand.

So why do so many bright school-leavers, with three good A-level passes tucked safely beneath their belts, *think* it worthwhile to embark on the longest and hardest undergraduate course on offer?

A medical qualification does carry with it benefits which will be obvious even to innocents unaware of most of the realities of the medical life. Doctors are, by and large, respected by their fellow citizens, and so entering the trade is one way of acquiring the kind of social status which most of us would like to enjoy. Doctors do exercise a considerable influence and even power over their clients and within the community, and that prospect must appeal to many. And, as Ellis Downes points out, a doctor need never be unemployed. Being a doctor also opens a way to many kinds of

widely differing careers, from becoming a tycoon in the pharmaceutical industry to transplanting livers in Cambridge, and from
editing the *Lancet* to caring for lepers in the African bush, so that all
manner of tastes and talents may be satisfied and deployed. But are
such attractions enough to explain and justify the choice of medicine
as a career?

A few students, like Bill Grove, may find themselves studying
medicine almost 'by accident'. More, like Ellis Downes, will have
chosen the profession because they have calculated that it does offer
an attractive mix of science, technology and human contact. I
suspect, however, that a majority are not guided by any such well-
defined purpose, but just have a gut feeling that they want to be
doctors. In other words, just like clergymen, and possibly teachers,
they feel a sense of vocation which can't be readily accounted for in
baldly rational terms.

In the days when I was engaged in the interviewing game I used to
take a somewhat mean line with the young hopefuls who told us that
they 'wanted to serve their fellow beings'. I'd point out that bankers,
dustmen, parsons, grocers and a host of other functionaries all serve
the needs of society and their fellows in an effective and essential
fashion, so why plump for medicine as their chosen approach to
achieving that end? The unfortunate children rarely had coherent
answers to that sneaky supplementary question (which was asked
not in order to embarrass them but because I had a genuine wish to
discover what was happening in their minds), but I never held that
against them, and was (and am) convinced that the presence of a
strong ambition to join the healing trade, even when it can't be
readily explained, is among the best of reasons for giving an
otherwise suitable candidate the chance.

But how are the 'otherwise suitable' to be identified? More than
that, with academically qualified applicants outnumbering available
places by something like ten to one, how do you identify the best?

Everybody I have spoken to agrees that a satisfactory answer to
that question has yet to be found, and that the present mechanisms
employed are at best inadequate and at worst an ill-conducted
lottery.

It is said that the late Henry Miller, when Dean of Medicine at the
University of Newcastle, did, indeed, select students by lot. Miller

was a famous 'character' who had small regard for the conventions and relished the pleasures of the flesh. So, believing that any task should be made as enjoyable as may be, he would organize a faculty champagne party during the course of which he'd produce a hat containing the names of all the year's applicants. The first 100 (or whatever) drawn were 'in', and the rest got letters of regret. The practice only ended when it was noised abroad and indignant protests flooded in. Apocryphal or not, the Miller method would probably prove as fair and effective as many another more serious approach.

According to Sir Robert Kilpatrick approximately half the UK medical schools judge candidates solely on their written records, and even though these do include 'a fair amount of opinion from their secondary schools' he favours the addition of an interview, since entrants should be chosen 'not just on intellectual but also on personality grounds'. But he concedes that 'the evidence for the discriminatory value of the interview is not high'. One problem is the lack of definition of the qualities required in a doctor, or a means of testing them.

Bill Grove remembers a 'controlled clinical trial' carried out in the USA a few years ago. For a period applicants to one medical school were selected entirely on their college examination results. Then the selectors switched to interviewing everybody and accepting people they thought would make 'nice doctors'. The two groups were assessed for their performance during their training, and there was no measurable difference between them. By the time they'd been churned through the mill they were all of a kind. 'So it probably makes no difference how you select them. The only question is whether the way you do it is fair to the applicants.'

Like me, Bill Grove believes that 'Perhaps, most importantly, you should try and gauge how much people want to be doctors, and perhaps it's the people who really want to be doctors who should be allowed in.' It's a superficially attractive solution to the problem, but, on his own testimony, Bill wouldn't be a doctor now if his inquisitors had concentrated on that issue. After all, he went into medicine 'almost by accident'.

But improving interview techniques and understandings is not enough. Wendy Savage says, 'I think we need to change the way we train doctors and change the way we select doctors, so that we don't just take in kids of eighteen who've done nothing but study very hard at school to get the requisite A-levels. In the States they can do a degree in a different discipline and then do a four-year medical course, and then, at the end of the day, they're just as technologically qualified as our people are. Why do we think that we have to take everybody in at eighteen?'

Her point is that the traditional UK method of moderating entry to the craft results in the inclusion of some of the least adequate and the exclusion of some of the most adequate potential medical practitioners. 'We should be selecting students because they've shown that they actually like people and are interested in providing care, perhaps because they've been social workers or physiotherapists, or whatever. Then at least we'd broaden the input and perhaps get away from this terrible domination of medicine by the professional middle classes.' A domination which, in that good woman's view, alienates the profession from the community it is supposed to serve.

David Owen says that 'We've set such a high academic threshold for doctors that we're in danger of losing the broader mind, and the broader balance, and the broader education. Medicine is not a pure science. It's a behavioural science. And in demanding the level of academic performance we now ask for we're losing some of the humanitarians, and this is very dangerous.'

I asked Joe Collier whether he could define the personal and intellectual qualities desirable in a doctor.

'When you're choosing future doctors you don't know those answers. I know what I want, and I think I know what patients want. Patients want somebody who listens – somebody obviously informed, somebody who seems to be interested and understanding, somebody prepared to be firm without being dominant, and somebody prepared to change and to be compassionate. A listening, compassionate, bothering person is a damned good start. The ability to change your mind is very valuable.'

Joe says that 'Nobody really knows what a good doctor is, and until we know what we want, and which eighteen-year-olds are going to produce what we want, we're stuck.'

There are tests available which purport to assess qualities such as compassion, adaptability and even honesty, and they might be usefully applied to school-leavers asking to enter medical school. At the Royal Free they have a couple of students sitting with the interviewing panel. The students don't vote, but can ask questions and voice opinions, and, being closer in age and (presumably) attitude to the probably overawed supplicants, they must add a valuable extra edge to the probing process.

Julia Neuberger believes that *all* candidates should be subjected to interviews designed by experts, and be assessed not just by doctors but also by, say, nurses and consumers. (She is very keen on more lay people becoming involved in all kinds of medical decision-making, including the way the profession runs itself. 'Having doctors and non-doctors working together makes for quite a good creative tension when it's done well. . . . The problem is getting the right sort of people, because they've got to be both trusted by the profession and sufficiently tough to speak out.')

There is general agreement that at least a year spent doing something completely different between leaving school and starting the course would broaden the mind wonderfully, and also help to sort out the determined from the not so sure, and that perhaps this should become a requirement, or at least be seen as an important plus when choosing the lucky 10 per cent.

Yet more effectively, the variety of talents and attitudes which medicine can use and needs could be mightily enhanced if entry requirements were far less rigid, and if a significant proportion of medical school places was reserved for mature students who had earned a degree in another subject or worked for a period of years in some other job (and not necessarily one of the other so-called caring professions). Certainly such candidates could be assumed to possess in high degree the all-important quality of commitment.

What is beyond doubt is that new, adventurous and well-informed approaches to the selection and training of doctors are urgently required if the profession is to prosper and render the best possible service to its customers – which is what it is, or should be, all about.

7   Tomorrow's Doctors

Will the NHS survive?

'I believe it's the greatest social experiment in history,' says John Marks. 'I believe it's as near the ideal way of providing health care as you'll get. And I think you'd have to look very hard and long now to find someone who disagreed. In fact in all the letters I've had – and I've had hundreds – I've had just one doctor who said, "I don't believe in the Health Service and it ought to be abolished."'

'People of my generation are just old enough to remember what it was like before. I qualified the day the NHS started, so I was a student under the old system. The old system couldn't cope with what it had then. It would *never* have coped with modern medicine. Not without beggaring people, like it does in the States.'

There seems no doubt that John Marks's assessment of popular and, indeed, expert feeling and opinion, is right, and that both the bulk of the medical profession and most of its customers would bitterly resist any attempt to turn the NHS into a skeleton of its present form, providing only a third-rate safety net for citizens unable to fund their own health needs.

But the fact that our Health Service is cherished by its functionaries and beneficiaries alike doesn't mean that doctors and their paramedical colleagues and the system within which they operate are immune to criticism.

Professor Bosanquet says that 'Being Minister of Health is now the most unpopular job in any country round the world. Twenty years ago being Minister of Labour was, but with changes in industrial relations that's now a much easier job. Ask the twenty most powerful people in any country to make a free association with the word "doctor". It's not with "healing" – it's with "costs", "aggravation", "lack of discipline", "lack of output".'

So doctors, it appears, no longer enjoy a high and virtuous reputation with politicians and other 'managers' of society. They still command public esteem, but, as we have seen, the consumers of medical care are also becoming ever more critical and demanding.

If the profession is to retain respect, and, perhaps more importantly from its own point of view, a reasonable degree of control over the manner in which it operates (if it wants to survive as a self-regulating profession), then doctors must be prepared to abandon or modify many of their traditional attitudes and practices, and, in particular, must accept the idea that they are only a part of society, and, indeed, only a part of the Health Service, and are not inhabiting 'an *Island*, entire of it self'. They must demonstrate that they are constantly striving to provide the best possible value for the vast sums of money which the practice of their craft absorbs, and they must show that they accept the fact that they are in business for the benefit of their clients and of society, and only incidentally for their own prosperity and satisfaction.

Keeping in Touch

To give value for money a doctor must remain competent and up-to-date. One hundred, or even fifty years ago, it was possible for a newly qualified doctor to imagine himself sufficiently knowledge-able to embark upon four or five decades of practice without any absolute need ever to look at another book or sit out another lecture. Today, advances in the understanding of disease, and the pace of production of entirely novel drugs and other forms of therapy, are so rapid that some form of continuing education is as essential to competence as a sound basic training.

There are now, throughout the country, postgraduate medical centres attached to hospitals where local general practitioners can attend seminars and lectures. Family doctors can earn extra payments for attending these and other approved events of an educational nature, but the organization of such opportunities tends to be on a pretty haphazard and free-wheeling basis. Often, for example, a consultant will be roped in to discourse upon some aspect of his specialty, but such chats may have little relevance to the practical problems faced daily in the surgery, and, at the sacrifice of a few extra pounds of income, a slothful or self-satisfied or hard-pressed practitioner can avoid such happenings altogether.

Doctors don't know nearly enough about the use of drugs, and this is the most serious deficiency in their professional competence. Joe Collier claims that, given the money, he could organize a team to compile and distribute a drug information tape a month to each of the nation's 70,000 prescribers, and he believes some such vigorous approach to the problem is essential, and that the Government should foot the bill. Certainly much more use could be made of the various powerful techniques of 'distance learning'.

But how do you persuade practitioners to use any instructional schemes on offer? Sir Robert Kilpatrick is sceptical about the efficacy of cash bribes but has great faith in the power of 'peer review' whereby doctors check up on one another's performance, and, given the provision of the means for continuing education (the easiest element of the campaign to achieve), he believes that a system and habit of medical audit designed and administered by the profession would be the right way to ensure that doctors do make the effort to use them and keep up-to-date.

The danger of losing touch is not confined to GPs, although they do work more in isolation than their hospital colleagues. The Royal Colleges have been busy organizing registers of those they consider qualified, by examination and experience, to practise the various specialties the colleges represent. Terence English suggests that in future achieving inclusion on such registers will not be an end to the matter, but that, every ten years, perhaps, the duly certified will have to demonstrate their fitness to remain on the list. Their performance will be reviewed, and they might also be required to demonstrate their knowledge and grasp of, say, the recent literature on their subject.

This would involve acknowledged experts judging their fellow acknowledged experts, so I asked Sir Terence English, 'Sed quis custodiet ipsos Custodes?', and had the impression that this tricky problem hadn't quite been ironed out. Senior Registrars, for example, often feel, and often with some justification, that they know a good deal more about the leading edges of their specialty than some of their official elders and betters. They have to, in order to maximize their chances of climbing the next and most competitive rung in Moran's ladder.

But, however it is done, it seems inevitable (and is certainly desirable) that doctors (just like airline pilots, but not judges or bishops) will be required to demonstrate throughout their working lives that they remain on top of the job, and are, indeed, giving value for money received, and that we are safe (or as safe as may be) in their hands.

It might even be that the panels empowered to decide whether a doctor remains worthy to receive a salary or contract from the State will include managers and consumers, and that, to remain employed, a member of the healing trade will be required to show that he matches up not only to the technical and clinical standards demanded by the princes of his profession, but also to the different but no less important standards of conduct and diligence demanded by his customers.

This is not far removed from the requirements for success in a free market. 'Going private' wouldn't make life any easier for most doctors, and most doctors know that, and they also know that 'going private' would significantly reduce their capacity to help people.

Paying Doctors

Dr Cracknell believes that within the next decade family doctors will become salaried employees of the State.

When the NHS was established, Aneurin Bevan would have been delighted to employ GPs as civil servants so that his Ministry could specify, in detail, their duties and terms of service. It didn't happen because GPs, represented by the BMA, insisted that they would only serve the new system if they remained 'independent', contracting their services, but staying out of State control.

This was a disastrous mistake on the GPs' part, for, as they soon discovered, when you contract to deliver a service for an agreed price you remain responsible for all the costs and hassles involved in fulfilling your contractual obligations. They found they couldn't provide a twenty-four-hour-a-day and 365-day-a-year service to their NHS customers for the reward offered and still make a decent living, and family doctoring became a thoroughly unpopular option with new graduates. So the Government, just to keep the all-important ship of primary care afloat, has had to add this and that

TOMORROW'S DOCTORS

extra payment and reimbursement for the services provided, but each extra payment has involved an extra obligation or additional paperwork. So GPs have found themselves directed and constrained in their activities to at least the same degree as a salaried employee is controlled, but without the advantage of having the boss responsible for the chore of providing and organizing all the tools of the trade, such as premises and telephones and secretaries and stationery and postage stamps, and also (most importantly) for arranging and funding out-of-hours and holiday cover. The new GP contract has further eroded the family doctor's always largely illusory 'independence', while actually increasing his administrative load.

The contractor status of family doctors has, in fact, proved highly advantageous to the Government, which has been able to run the general medical services through the agency of Family Health Services Authorities (the old FPCs), employing a comparatively small staff, and, in Dr Cracknell's words, 'an enormous new bureaucracy' would be needed to administer a salaried service. But, he believes, GPs, increasingly unhappy with the burdensome nature of their contracts, will recognize and demand the many advantages of a salaried status, and, if they don't get it, will start voting with their feet.

What Next?

Tomorrow's doctors will be better educated by means of an undergraduate curriculum which will fit them to be not just competent medical technicians but informed and understanding members of the society they serve.

The academically and scientifically inclined will continue to 'push back the frontiers of knowledge', and their efforts must be supported and sustained, but they will no longer be regarded as the leaders of their profession just because they know a lot about a very little.

General practice will become the major instrument for the delivery of medical care, and GPs will provide more and more of the technical services now centred in hospitals.

New technology will give them the ability to do more and more for their customers' physical symptoms and complaints, but, says

143

Professor Bosanquet, 'Until doctors are willing to go back to being doctors of the mind as well as of the body – of the whole person – they will continue to lose credibility.'

Exactly so.

Index